The Maudsley Handbook of Practical Psychiatry

Fourth Edition

OXFORD MEDICAL PUBLICATIONS

The Maudsley Handbook of Practical Psychiatry

Fourth Edition

edited by
David Goldberg
Institute of Psychiatry, Denmark Hill, London
and
Robin Murray
Institute of Psychiatry, Denmark Hill, London

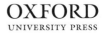

OXFORD
UNIVERSITY PRESS

OXFORD

UNIVERSITY PRESS

Great Clarendon Street, Oxford OX2 6DP

Oxford University Press is a department of the University of Oxford.
It furthers the University's objective of excellence in research,
scholarship, and education by publishing worldwide in

Oxford   New York
Auckland   Bangkok   Buenos Aires   Cape Town   Chennai
Dar es Salaam   Delhi   Hong Kong   Istanbul   Karachi   Kolkata
Kuala Lumpur   Madrid   Melbourne   Mexico City   Mumbai   Nairobi
São Paulo   Shanghai   Taipei   Tokyo   Toronto

Oxford is a registered trade mark of Oxford University Press
in the UK and in certain other countries

Published in the United States
by Oxford University Press Inc., New York

© Oxford University Press, 2002

A catalogue record for this title is available from the British Library

Library of Congress Cataloging in Publication Data
(Data available)

ISBN 0 19 851609 6 [Flexicover]

10 9 8 7 6 5 4 3 2 1

Typeset by Cepha Imaging Pvt Ltd, India

Printed on acid-free paper
in China

Preface

Robin Murray, Professor of Psychiatry, joins Sir David Goldberg as an Editor of this edition of *The Maudsley Handbook of Practical Psychiatry*. Since publishing the last edition, this book has been translated into Italian, Japanese, Russian, and Spanish. We are delighted that a book written for trainees in the UK has been found useful in other countries, and aware of a heavy burden upon us to keep the book up to date. As we go to press, the Mental Health Act has yet to be revised; we have therefore continued to describe the present law, but have written a short section on likely future changes.

Once more, we have leaned heavily on others as consultant advisers, and have relied upon our trainees to tell us what they want to see in a handbook to be carried in their pocket or bag. The trainees have read every word of the text, and made helpful comments throughout. Many sections have been completely rewritten, and other sections have been added since the last edition. We are very grateful to those of our consultant colleagues who have produced or rewritten text for us: in particular: Jonathon Bindman, Dinesh Bughra, George Szmukler, Mike Crowe, Rob Kerwin, Clive Meux, Declan Murphy, Siobhan Murphy, Eric Taylor, and Ann Ward.

The trainees who assisted us were Drs Elvira Bramon, Matt Broome, Dr James McCabe, Lucy Cameron, Steve Church, Paola Dazzan, Elaine Healy, Clare Henderson, Tennyson Lee, Paul Moran, Carmine Pariente, Marco Picchioni, Rob Stewart, Nigel Tunstall, Elizabeth Walsh, and Harvey Wickham. Our profound thanks go to all who assisted with the task, and apologies to those whose text was modified or not used. As Editors, we must accept sole responsibility for deciding what is to appear in this book.

D. G.
R. M.

The Maudsley Hospital
August 2002

Contents

List of abbreviations

AIDS	acquired immune deficiency syndrome
AMTS	Abbreviated Mental Test Score
ASW	Approved Social Worker
AUDIT	Alcohol Use Disorders Identification Test
BMI	body mass index
CAN	Camberwell Assessment of Needs
CBT	cognitive behavioural therapy
CNS	central nervous system
CPA	care programme approach
CPN	community psychiatric nurse
CSA	child sexual abuse
CSF	cerebrospinal fluid
CJD	Creutzfeld–Jakob disease
CT	computed tomography
CVA	cerebrovascular accident
CYP	cytochrome oxidase
DSH	deliberate self-harm
DSM-IV	Diagnostic and Statistical Manual IV
DTF	Drug Tariff Formula
DTs	delirium tremens
ECG	electrocardiography
ECT	electroconvulsive therapy
EEG	electroencephalography
EPSE	extrapyramidal side-effects
ESR	erythrocyte sedimentation rate
GABA	gamma-aminobutyric acid
GP	general practitioner
HIV	human immunodeficiency virus
HRT	hormone replacement therapy
ICD-10	International Classification of Diseases, 10th edition
ICU	intensive care unit
IgG	immunoglobulin G
IM	intramuscular

IMHP	intramuscular high potency
IV	intravenous
IVHP	intravenous high potency
LFT	liver function test
LSD	lysergic acid diethylamide
MAOI	monoamine oxidase inhibitor
MDMA	methylene dioxymethamphetamine
ME	myalgic encephalopathy
MHRT	Mental Health Review Tribunal
MMSE	Mini-mental State Examination
MND	motor neuron disease
MRI	magnetic resonance imaging
MS	multiple sclerosis
MSE	mental state examination
NHS	National Health Service
NMS	neuroleptic malignant syndrome
OCP	oral contraceptive pill
PD	Parkinson's disease
PET	positron emission tomography
PTA	post-traumatic amnesia
RBC	red blood cell count
RMO	Responsible Medical Officer
SLE	systemic lupus erythematosus
SPECT	single-photon emission computed tomography
SSRI	selective serotonin reuptake inhibitor
TCA	tricyclic antidepressant
TFT	thyroid function test
TPHA	*Treponema pallidum* haemagglutination (test)
VDRL	Venereal Disease Research Laboratory (test)
WBC	white blood cell count
WHO	World Health Organization

The psychiatric interview with adults

This chapter separates the kinds of interview techniques that are usual when making a full assessment of a patient (see below) from those required while on emergency duty (p. 8). There are special considerations when interviewing elderly patients (p. 11) or those with a learning disability (p. 14).

Interviews on the wards or outpatient department with adult patients

The psychiatric interview has in common many features to that of the medical interview—namely that its two main goals are to elicit the necessary information to make a diagnosis and to try to understand the aetiology of that disorder for that particular individual (the 'formulation'). Again, as in medicine, most of the information required for a diagnosis in psychiatry comes from the history rather than the examination or any investigations. However, there is a third feature to the psychiatric assessment that, although important in medicine, is more explicit in the psychiatric setting: using the interview as a means to obtain a therapeutic trusting relationship with the patient. This is particularly important when the patient may not feel they have a problem, either due to a psychotic illness or where they have considerable ambivalence about their desire for help with their problems—such as eating disorders or substance abuse. This approach, whereby the patient's problems are reviewed against the backdrop of offers of psychiatric help, has been formalized as compliance therapy and motivational enhancement therapy. Lastly, the psychiatric interview can also have value as a psychotherapeutic intervention.

Recording information elicited from the interview

Notes are best written at the time of the interview, remembering to name and date each sheet and to give the time of the interview on the first sheet, because it is rare that the busy clinician will have time to write up notes after meetings. Some doctors find it helpful to record information under different headings on several sheets at once; this is particularly useful when recording verbatim examples of speech for the mental state. Before the interview, any referral letters and past medical notes should be reviewed, and any confusion should be clarified or further information requested.

Outside the interview room

After introducing yourself, explain who you are and why you wish to see the patient. If relatives are present, ask them whether there is anything they that feel you should know before seeing the patient, and explain that they will have an opportunity to speak to you after the interview. Generally it is best to see adult patients alone.

In the interview room

Reintroduce yourself to the patient, as many will forget or mishear your name and you will want to use this as part of your cognitive assessment later. Explain the purpose of the interview and say how much time you expect to have available. Explain that you need to write some notes, but say that they are a confidential record. (If the assessment is for medicolegal purposes, it should clearly be stated that what is said in the interview will be put in a report that may be given to third parties or placed before the court. In this situation the patient should be asked to consent in writing). Generally it is advisable to avoid lengthy interviews and best to collect full information over a number of days.

History of presenting complaint

The main reasons for taking a history and performing the mental state examination can get lost when starting out in psychiatry—not least because the chaos of many of patients is reflected in their presentation and in the telling of their story. Remember that you are taking the history and assessing the mental state so that you can make an assessment that helps you plan management. This assessment goes further than making an accurate ICD-10 diagnosis, although this is crucial.

You essentially want to answer the question, 'Why has this patient presented in this way at this point in time', in order to form a management plan that really fits your patient's needs.

Start your interview with an open question, such as, 'What have you come to see me about?' or 'Are there any concerns that your family have about you?' Do not write anything down yet—you should be looking at the patient and listening to them. Only start to write after you have heard the patient's current symptoms and have established the order in which the various complaints developed. Write an account in chronological order, giving the duration of each complaint or problem. This account of the evolution of the patient's problems should include the social milieu within which they developed, highlighting any key precipitating events. The patient's symptoms and attributions (what the patient thinks caused the symptom) should be described, as well as how he or she tried to cope with the experience. The effects of any treatment taken should be noted. The effect of the patient's symptoms on their social,occupational, interpersonal (family, marriage, sexual functioning, responsibility) functioning and self-care (including eating, sleeping, weight, excretory functions, and substance use) should be described.

Precipitants

These may not have emerged in the patient's spontaneous account of precipitants and it is worthwhile screening for these, again because it informs management plans:

- Any life events (or anniversaries of life events)
- Alcohol or drug misuse
- Non-adherence to medications if any has been prescribed.

Suicidal thoughts and actions

This topic is dealt with more fully in Chapter 8 (pp. 106–9).

The questions form a natural hierarchy, which is followed as far as necessary:

- Do you feel that you have a future?
- Do you feel that life's not worth living?
- Do you ever feel completely hopeless?
- Do you ever feel you'd be better of dead and away from it all?
- Have you made any plans? (If overdose, have you handled the tablets?)
- Have you ever made an attempt to take your own life?
- What prevents you from doing so?
- Have you made any arrangements for your affairs after your death?

For other special topics, such as alcohol and drug problems, eating disorders, sexual disorders, epilepsy and other organic problems, also see Chapter 8.

Life charts
It is often helpful to relate events in the patient's life to illnesses that he
or she has had. Life charts are especially valuable if the patient has
both a physical illness and psychological problems; the column headings should then be age, life event, physical illness, and psychological
illness. The 'physical illness' column may, of course, be omitted if there
is nothing to record.

In its simplest form, there is a line on the life chart for each year of
the patient's life, but it may be more informative to use a non-linear
timescale and to give more space to some key periods of the patient's
life, and less to others.

When you have finished taking the history of the present complaint,
recapitulate this history back to the patient; ask, 'Is that right?' and
'Is there anything else I should ask you?' At this stage, go on to the
mental state (see Ch. 4, p. 60).

Family history

The amount of detail recorded will be influenced by the nature of the
patient's illness. It is helpful to draw a picture of the patient's family,
using squares for males and circles for females. Enter the first name
against the symbol for the sib. Those who have died are indicated by
an oblique line through the circle or square, together with date of
death and cause of death. Marriages ended by divorce are indicated by
a double oblique line. For an example, see Fig. 1.1.

You draw this figure with the patient's assistance, and in full view.
Then ask, 'Has anyone in your family suffered from a mental illnesses?'
and, if so, enter details against them. This is the most informative
way of collecting information about genetic loading (see also p. 25).
If parents have separated, indicate on the family tree the age of the
patient at the time when the separation occurred. Also ask regarding
alcohol and suicide history in family members.

Personal history

This should not be a mechanical procedure, but an opportunity to
test ideas about the patient's life, depending upon the nature of
their current problems. Test hypotheses about the patient, using a
'negotiating' style: 'I wonder whether…'

Family background
Ask the patient to describe his or her parents or step-parents: what
were they like, how did the patient get on with each of them? Where
does the patient come in the sibship, and what are the achievements
of each sib? Try to make a determination of the *family atmosphere*.
What was the general experience of being a child in that family;
were they happy times? (If not, what was the problem?) Elicit
early childhood difficulties and general development. (See also
Ch. 3, p. 39).

Childhood
Place of birth and birth difficulties. Who brought the patient up and where; occupation of parents or care-giver, general nature and quality of relationship with each. (See pp. 16–17)

School
Age of leaving school and qualifications. How did the patient get on with teachers and other students? What were the patient's best subjects? How did the patient get on with teachers and other students? Was the patient bullied? Did he or she truant?

Occupational history
Age at first job, general areas of employment, periods of unemployment and why. Frequency of job change. Current job: enjoyable, any problems? (This provides an opportunity to judge whether the patient realized his or her potential; whether the patient has persistence. Frequent changes of job, or leaving many jobs without good reason, suggest an abnormal personality.)

Psychosexual history
Current 'partner', time with that person, difficulties; is the partner supportive? Previous partners. Age at first girlfriend/boyfriend (ask directly about both same and opposite sexual relationships). Age at puberty and first sexual experience. Any unwanted sexual experiences? Any unsafe sex? If patient has steady partner, ask about the relationship. Any children (details)? (See pp. 20, 114–17 for fuller details.)

Past psychiatric history
Illnesses, admissions, treatment and episodes of self-harm.

Past and current medical and surgical history
Co-morbid physical illness is common in older patients and must be assessed comprehensively. All current medication, both regular and 'as required' should be documented. A collateral history from the patient's general practitioner may be helpful. The patient's view of their own health may be an important feature in their presenting complaint.

Alcohol use
All patients should be asked about their alcohol consumption. Screening aims to detect whether an alcohol problem is present and, if so, whether it is likely to respond to brief intervention or to require specialized treatment. Some commonly used screening questions are derived from the Alcohol Use Disorders Identification Test (AUDIT; see Appendix 1):

- How often do you have a drink containing alcohol?
- How many drinks containing alcohol do you have on a typical day when you are drinking?
- How often do you have six or more drinks on one occasion?

Illustrative family tree

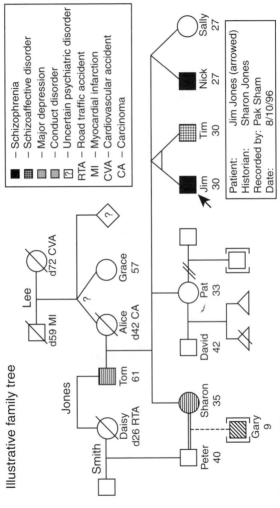

Figure 1.1 Illustrative family tree.

List of symbols used in family trees

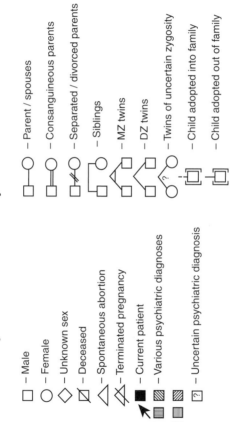

Figure 1.1 (continued)

These questions can be made less threatening by being incorporated into an assessment of general health/lifestyle or into the medical history.

Drug misuse

All patients should be asked about their use of illicit or over-the-counter drugs. However, for most patients a few brief screening questions will suffice; for example:

- Are there any other tablets or medicines that you take, apart from those you get from your doctor?
- Is there anything you buy from the chemists or get from friends?
- Have you used any (illegal) drugs such as ... amphetamines/speed, ecstasy, cocaine/crack, LSD/acid or heroin?
- What about tablets to settle your nerves or to help you sleep (such as temazepam or diazepam)?

Medication

Current medication. Any allergies or problems with medication.

Forensic history

Ever been trouble with the law or had points on your driving licence? If so, record full details. Record name of current Probation Officer (if relevant).

Social history

Accommodation, finances, home activities, outside activities, carers (For fuller details, see Ch. 2, pp. 27–9.)

Premorbid personality

Before you became unwell, what were you like? Prompt patient for whether they had many friends; could they trust people; what their temper was like; how they coped with life; how they dealt with criticism; were they very tidy? (Remember that information from an informant about personality is even more valuable than that from the patient, whose views may be influenced by the current illness. For more details, see pp. 19.)

Interviews on emergency duty

The assessment while on emergency duty is likely to be much more focused on the presenting problem than the fuller assessments carried out on the wards.

Background information including the referral

Obtaining background information will enhance the efficiency and effectiveness of the assessment as well as promoting greater safety, but lays the clinician open to bias. In most situations, information is usually limited and in the form of a letter. Background information becomes particularly important in the context of the psychiatric emergency.

The commonest psychiatric examination the trainee will have to undertake is the emergency assessment in the hospital setting.

Typically the patient will be heralded by a telephone call. For each call the following details should be elicited and recorded clearly in the notes, remembering that this may be the only opportunity to obtain some of the information.

- The name of the referrer and who they are in relation to the patient.
- How you can contact them again should you wish to.
- The patient's name and address (including postcode).
- General details, including referrer's concerns.

At this stage, before accepting the referral, if you are in doubt about whether or not the patient falls within your remit, explain this to the referring agent and arrange to call them back with the details (including telephone number) of the correct institution.

Then ask the referrer for details of why they wish to send this patient to you both in terms of their concerns regarding the patient and how they feel the patient should or might be helped. If the referral is a result of unusual behaviour, record a detailed account of who observed what.

This is particularly important for patients who are brought by the police (e.g. under a section 136), as this may be the only objective, collaborative information available on the patient and the only opportunity to elicit and record it.

Where the referrer is a healthcare professional, obtain as much information as possible. This can be grouped into:

- Physical health problems (past and current including medication).
- Mental health problems (past, current assessment and medication).
- Risk to self and to others (past and current).

Agree with the referrer where and when the patient will be seen.

Preparation of the room

The practical aspects of eliciting and recording information should be considered: quiet, well lit, private, with a writing surface. Typically the optimal seating arrangement is at an angle of 45–90°, for example around one corner of a desk. Safety issues must always be considered routinely before seeing every patient; these include (see also Ch. 7, p. 98):

- Never sit the patient so that you are hemming them in. The furniture should be so arranged that it is easy for either of you to leave.
- Remove any object from sight that might be used as a weapon, for example letter openers or large paperweights. In a volatile situation, the act of sighting a potential weapon can catalyse decompensation into violence.
- If there is a panic button in the room, know where it is, how it works and whether or not it will summon aid after hours. If there is no panic button, know how to summon help.
- Avoid using rooms that are in an isolated area.

- Inform nursing colleagues about what you are doing and how long you expect to be.
- If you believe that there is more than usual risk, arrange for correspondingly greater numbers of (nursing) colleagues in increasing proximity. Before the interview discuss your concerns and how to manage an unwanted event.

Assessments on emergency duty

The work is of necessity problem focused, with only those aspects of the history and examination that are necessary to understand the nature of the patient's present problems. Thus, the history of the present symptoms and a focused mental state examination are essential, as well as detailed enquiry about drugs and medications taken (or not taken) recently. Previous psychiatric history should be covered briefly, and an effort made to collect information from others who may be accompanying the patient.

The doctor will wish to admit all those whose illness represents a threat to themselves or to others, unless satisfactory alternative care arrangements are available. Readmissions of psychotic patients can sometimes be prevented if the key worker is available, or if resources permit a very brief stay in a community hostel while medication is resumed.

Interviews in outpatients

Forming a management plan

It may be necessary to complete your information by gathering from other sources before entering this stage of the assessment. If a relative is available, ask the patient whether he or she minds whether you see them. (A parent of a child under 16 years of age has a legal right to see you, but patients over the age of 16 can object.) Use your judgment about whether to have the relative in the room while the management plan is communicated to the patient. Other things being equal, it is usually to be preferred, as the relative's attitude to what you propose is likely to be a critical factor in determining compliance, and the patient may not remember everything that you say.

Ask the patient how they expected that you would help them. If their expectations sound reasonable, give them details of what you think would be the best course and ask them whether that sounds reasonable to them.

If their expectations are quite different from your own, explain your reasons for preferring a different course of action. The relative is often very useful at this point, if present. Give your advice in small quantities, and get the patient to agree with what you are saying.

If the patient needs an **investigation**, explain why, what it will involve, and what steps the patient needs to take to get it done. If you are referring them to a colleague, tell them your colleague's name and explain why you wish the patient to see them.

If you are **prescribing a drug**, say, 'The drug I usually use for your problem is [name of drug]. Have you heard of that? (If they have, have they ever been prescribed it, and did it help?) Tell them:

- The main effects of the drug.
- Its side-effects.
- The length of time for which they are likely to have to take it.
- Whether the drug is habit-forming.

If you are suggesting a **course of therapeutic interviews**, say:

- How many interviews, and how long each will last.
- What the purpose of the interviews will be.
- What you expect the patient to discuss during them.

Get the patient to agree to the plan, or you may well have been wasting your time.

Assessment of the elderly patient

This is essentially the same as that of younger adults, but there are differences of emphasis that need consideration. Assessment is frequently complicated by the patient's **intellectual impairment, physical ill-health** including hearing and visual disability, and **clouding of consciousness.** As a consequence it may be necessary to carry out the assessment over several sessions and essential to obtain a **collateral history** from a close relative or carer. Nowadays, the initial assessment will usually be carried out in the patient's own home.

Old age psychiatry is largely concerned with four major diagnoses: dementia, delirium, depression and delusional disorder (including schizophrenia). Clearly, neuroses, personality disorders and substance abuse do occur in the elderly but, to simplify what follows, discussion will be limited to the four diagnostic groups listed above.

History of presenting complaint

Bear in mind that some patients with dementia or delirium may lack insight. Also, direct questioning about memory function may be helpful:

- Do you have any difficulty with your memory?
- Do you forget where you have left things more than you used to?
- Do you think your memory is worse than that of other people of your age?

Other cognitive problems, such as dysphasia, dyspraxia and agnosia, should be asked about (see pp. 71, 75).

Elderly patients may not admit to feeling 'depressed' or 'low in spirits'; careful questioning as to other depressive symptoms, such as suicidal ideas, diurnal variation, low self-esteem, hopelessness, guilt, insomnia, anorexia and weight loss, will assist in making the diagnosis.

- Paranoid or psychotic features may need to be elicited directly:
- Do you get on well with your neighbours or have you had any difficulty with them?
- Do you ever hear or see things that other people do not? Are people spying on you or plotting against you?
- Are people stealing from you?

Many patients with dementia present to psychiatric services because of associated psychotic, affective or behavioural disturbances, rather than the cognitive problems. **These are best elicited from an informant.** Common psychotic symptoms in dementia include:

- Delusions of theft, persecution.
- Auditory and visual hallucinations.
- Misidentification syndromes.

Common behavioural problems include:

- Wandering.
- Aggression.
- Urinary incontinence.
- Elements of the Kluver–Bucy syndrome (i.e. binge eating, hyperorality, sexual disinhibition, misrecognition, rages, apathy, and hypermetamorphosis).

Ask whether symptoms had a sudden or gradual onset; the order in which symptoms developed is sometimes important, for instance in differentiating depression with cognitive impairment from 'real' dementia, of differentiating between different types of dementia.

Cognitive assessment

Most older people have no objections to cognitive assessment when it is introduced with tact. It is helpful to start off by asking whether the patient has experienced any problems with memory and concentration and, if so, whether this has bothered them and what sort of things they find they forget. After this, the cognitive assessment may make more sense. A common preamble used in research instruments is: 'I am going to ask a few questions about memory and concentration. Some of these questions may seem very easy and others might be quite difficult, but we need to ask everyone the same questions.'

Where the patient permits formal testing, a short cognitive screening test such as the Abbreviated Mental Test or the Mini-Mental State Examination (MMSE) may be used (see Appendix 2). For patients known to have dementia, the MMSE is helpful in giving an approximate idea of the severity of impairment. A high score may provide evidence against substantial cognitive impairment. It may also be helpful in future assessments to have an idea of previous function (and therefore it is important that previous assessments are accessed where possible to put any current score in context). It is vital to take previous education, levels of literacy, and sensory deficits into account when interpreting scores from these screening tests. For example, someone with high educational attainment may have clinically evident dementia and still achieve a maximum score on the MMSE. In addition, both screening tests have poor cross-cultural validity and results should be interpreted with appropriate caution.

Cognitive screening tests such as the MMSE provide relatively little information concerning specific cognitive deficits. Memory impairment cannot, for example, be adequately assessed through the recall of three words. Frontal lobe function is also poorly assessed by this instrument. If cognitive impairment is suspected, a formal assessment should be carried out as outlined in Chapter 5.

Family history

Specifically, a history in first-degree relatives of:

- Dementia, Parkinson's disease, mental illness.
- Heart or stroke disease, hypertension.
- Cancer, including leukaemia.
- Down's syndrome.

Personal history

Traumatic experiences occurring during war time (or at other times) that still bother the patient or cause distress. Sexual activity should be asked about in a straightforward and direct way. It should not be assumed that sexual behaviour will have ceased simply because a person is old.

Ask about reaction to life events:

- Retirement.
- Bereavement.
- Serious illness in the patient or a close relative.

Elder abuse is increasingly recognised. A series of neutral questions may allow further exploration of this difficult area:

- Has anyone shouted or insulted you recently?
- Has anyone hit you or handled you roughly recently?
- Has anyone stopped you getting the help you need recently?

Social history

This follows the usual schema outlined in Chapter 2 (pp. 27–9); however, important areas in the elderly, other than housing and finance, include:

- **Social network**—what support is there from family/friends, clubs; what day centres are attended, how frequently?
- **Home-care support**—does the patient receive meals-on-wheels, home helps and district nurses; how frequently, are they helpful?

Lastly, an account of the patient's ability to perform activities of daily living should be obtained. This should include information on the following:

- **Mobility**—the use of walking aids, whether stairs can be climbed without help.
- **Personal hygiene**—washing, continence, using the toilet, and dressing (e.g. Can you wash yourself without help? Do you have trouble controlling your bladder? Can you dress yourself without help?)
- **Domestic activities**—cooking, laundry, housework, and paying bills.

Taking a collateral history

Attempts should be made to obtain a collateral history for all psychiatric assessments. In the case of older patients, the following information may be obtained most accurately from an informant:

- History of cognitive decline.
- Onset and course of cognitive decline, if suspected.
- Personality change (suggestive of frontal lobe pathology).
- Behavioural disturbance associated with cognitive decline (see History of presenting complaint).
- Activities of daily living and level of support (see Social history).
- In the presence of confabulation, ascertaining deficits in long-term memory as part of the mental state examination may be impossible to establish without an informant.

In the collateral history, it is particularly important to investigate the extent of carer strain. This may be a component in the patient's presentation, is an important risk factor for elder abuse, and may affect later treatment decisions and prognosis.

Assessing patients with a learning disability

People with a mild learning disability can usually provide their own history; additional history from an informant is usually needed when the patient is moderately or severely disabled.

Remember that learning disability is not in itself an emergency; it is a permanent condition. Learning disability does not protect against the development of other conditions.

Always obtain information on the nature and duration of any recent changes, particularly behavioural changes: the opportunity to obtain this information from a **key informant** may not arise again.

In a genuine emergency, usually some **additional condition** has developed; this may be either physical or mental.

- Always eliminate **pain** as a cause for an acute behavioural disturbance: pain may arise from a life-threatening condition.

- Ask about recent **seizures** or other epileptic phenomena.

If diagnosis of learning disability is in doubt, ask the informant:

- Was this person's development delayed in childhood?
- Did this person attend a special school?
- Did they learn to read and write?
- What jobs has this person held?
- Is this person losing any skills?
- Does anyone in the family have a learning disability or developmental abnormality?

Terminating the interview

Tell the patient what you are going to do (e.g. write to their doctor, discuss their case with a colleague) and when they will next be hearing from the hospital or, in the case of an inpatient, when they will next be seeing you. You may not know exactly when you will be available to see a ward patient, and in that case give them some idea; for example, 'I'm next here on Thursday and I'll try to see you for half an hour during the afternoon'. If they are in outpatients, give them an appointment card with an identifying number on it. If you expect the patient to do anything, make sure this has been clearly understood by either the patient or their relative.

2

Special assessments with adults

Assessing early life experience

In the absence of a suitable informant, the patient may be able to report only what they have been told about their early years—the period of normal childhood amnesia. If they report amnesia for most of their childhood, there must be a strong suspicion that there have been events too painful to remember that have been actively obliterated. Significant events that will probably have influenced the person's early development, coping strategies, personality, relationship patterns and vulnerabilities are as follows:

1. Puerperal illness of the mother, leading to actual separation or subtle deficiencies in early maternal care.

2. Siblings born in rapid succession: pregnancy can interfere with a mother's ability to be receptive to her infant's hostility towards its unborn sibling. This can lead to suppression of feelings of rivalry and jealousy in the child, mistakenly reported as lack of jealousy.

3. Twinship stresses mother, twins and all the family. Rivalry between twins and their separate development may be obliterated in many ways, if parents find it too painful and complex to deal with. Its reported absence is abnormal.

4. Death of a parent and bereavement reactions of the survivors can have a lasting effect. Who helped the subject to mourn?

5. Chronic illness, especially mental illness of a parent. Was it a family secret? What help did the family have from outside? Who became the 'parental child'?

6. Parental strife and separation, which inevitably leads to divided loyalties. A mother who cannot separate from a violent partner exposes her children to confusion. They want to but cannot protect her, and they cannot understand why she does not leave to protect herself.

7. Single parenthood: poverty, lack of emotional support, frequent changes of sexual partner, increased risk of child abuse by partners.

8. Frequent changes of domicile: ruptures peer relationships and disrupts schooling.

9. Bullying at school suggests poor self-esteem, poor social skills, and insecure early attachment pattern.

10. Frequent hospitalizations: separations, painful operations, disruption, schooling and peer relations, over-anxious or disengaged parents.

11. Major environmental failure: in and out of care, foster homes, children's homes, childhood sexual and physical abuse, neglect, emotional deprivation.

Memories of sexual abuse

There is now compelling evidence from well conducted case–control studies that sexual abuse during childhood ('CSA') is followed by higher rates of depression and anxiety during childhood and early adult life, by a greater incidence of deliberate self-harm, and by eating disorders during adolescence and early adult life. As sexual abuse of children is commonly accompanied by both physical abuse and poor care, it is difficult to disentangle the specific ill-effects of each kind of abuse. However, not all patients who give vivid descriptions of sexual abuse have in fact been abused, and false memories are especially likely to occur after misguided 'therapeutic' efforts to recover such memories. The situation is complicated by the fact that some people who were actually abused have repressed their memories of the abuse, a fact that leads some self-styled therapists to embark on treatment designed to recover such memories.

Absent memories: amnesia for abuse

Children who presented for medical care following sexual abuse were seen as adults, on average, 17 years later. Over a third (38%) appeared to have no memory of their early abuse. Loss of memory was most common if the abuse occurred when they were young and was perpetrated by someone they knew.

Recovered false memories

'Recovered memories' are typically reported in the course of therapies that employ memory recovery techniques, including hypnosis (especially hypnotic regression), guided imagery, guided meditation and the use of so-called 'truth drugs'. Therapists practising these techniques state that the memories occur in the context of amnesia at the start of therapy, such that clients giving their life history would not be aware of abuse as a child.

False beliefs and inaccurate memories

There is a great deal of evidence for incorrect memories, that is where an event has happened but the details are recalled wrongly. This is because of the mental processing, some of it unconscious, that occurs when memories are recollected. The extent to which this occurs is outside the individual's awareness. There is an unstable relationship between confidence and accuracy.

Normal memory

To a degree, all memories are unreliable. They are not held like video tapes in the mind to be replayed at recall. Rather, when a memory is cued it is processed even prior to the stage at which it reaches awareness. This processing can include the incorporation of general knowledge or material from another record. After the remembering, information will be stored as a record of the remembering. The next time the cycle of remembering is entered, the recall may be for the original or may be for the previous recall. Not every detail of an event is stored in memory. When an event is recalled, it might need elaborating before it is intelligible to consciousness. What we are conscious of is a mixture of reproduction and reconstruction. Reconstructive memory is characterized by conflation of different events, filling out of detail and importation of information. Nothing can be recalled accurately from before the first birthday and little from before the second. Poor memory from before the fourth birthday is normal.

Factors that influence the degree of reconstruction include:

- the personal significance of the event
- its emotive content
- the time elapsed between the event occurring and its recall
- the age at which the event occurred
- the reasons why the person is remembering the event and the circumstances of recall.

Psychiatric practice and memories of sexual abuse

Obtaining a psychiatric history that may include sexual abuse poses difficulties. Repeated admissions to psychiatric hospitals leads to the history being recounted on many occasions. What we know about memory is that if there is extensive rehearsal of an imagined event the person can believe the event happened. The memory can become highly detailed and vivid to the person. The event can be altered in matters of detail by suggestion and leading questions. It is common practice for the patient's account to be recorded in psychiatric notes without any attempt to question the source or reliability of the memory. Indeed the American Psychiatric Association report stated:

> psychiatrists should maintain *an empathic, non judgmental, neutral stance* towards memories of sexual abuse. As in the treatment of all patients, care must be taken to avoid prejudging the cause of the patient's difficulties or the veracity of the patient's reports. A strong belief by the psychiatrist that sexual abuse, or other factors, are or are not the cause of the patient's problems is likely to interfere with appropriate assessment and treatment. Many individuals who have experienced sexual abuse have a history of not being believed by their parents, or others in whom they have put their trust. Expression of disbelief is likely to cause the patient further pain and decrease his/her willingness to seek psychiatric treatment. Similarly clinicians should not exert pressure on patients to believe in events that may have not occurred, or to prematurely disrupt important relationships or make other important decisions based on these speculations.

One of the strongest criteria in assessing the reliability of a memory is the accuracy with which it is anchored in place and time. However, it may be difficult to establish these sorts of fact in the context of the approach (empathic, non-judgmental) defined above. Thus, the history from the patient may be unreliable and the process of medical treatment may further contribute to faulty recollection.

The mental state and inaccuracies of memory

Abnormal mental states are likely to lead to errors in the reconstruction of memories. This is obvious in psychotic states but also occurs in extreme emotional states. In such states of mind there are errors and biases in memory processing, evaluative judgments and overall information processing.

Informants

The fact that memories can be unreliable is recognized in psychiatry and is why informants are often used to corroborate the history. This is recognized as good psychiatric practice. The history should be compiled from information elicited both from the patient and from one or more informants. The informant's account will not only amplify the patient's report of factual detail but will supplement the patient's account. Clinicians bear a heavy responsibility to do no harm. The desire to help the victims of childhood abuse heal is more than justified, but clinicians are urged to reflect upon the damage done by false accusations. Accepting the truth of what appear to be long forgotten memories elicited by therapy without corroboration can seriously injure and disrupt the lives of innocent people. For this reason, many psychiatrists feel uncomfortable if they attempt to get corroboration in this area. They are uncertain what questions they should ask and of whom. Are they not breaking confidentiality if they attempt to do this?

The corroborative evidence that is useful in a psychiatric history is different from that required for forensic reasons. Open, broad questions can be used. For example, if there is a history of CSA it would be reasonable to ask the parents, other relatives, and schools whether any difficulties or concerns were noted during the child's development.

Sexual disorders and couple relationship problems

Sexual history

- Age at puberty (voice breaking, shaving, menarche).
- Age at which first ejaculation occurred.
- Age at first masturbation. How was this regarded? Fantasies? Anxieties?
- Attitudes of parents to sexual matters.
- Sexual seduction or childhood sexual abuse?
- Any unusual sexual preferences? Fantasies? Activities?
- Homosexual or heterosexual orientation (fantasies, desires and experiences)?
- Any gender dysphoria, including non-arousing cross-dressing?
- Previous sexual experiences and relationships including painful or traumatic ones.
- Current sex life (if any)—marital, extramarital, visiting or cohabiting?
- Current frequency of masturbation?
- Level of sexual drive—any changes during this illness?
- Contraception? Safe sex? Sexually transmitted diseases?
- Sexual dysfunctions—desire, arousal or orgasm? Partner satisfied?
- Discrepancy in sexual interest between partners.
- Menopause? Hysterectomy? Hormone replacement?

Marital and relationship history

- Age at first intercourse.
- Number of previous engagements or serious relationships.
- Difficulties in these and reasons for break up.
- Age at present marriage (or cohabitation)—reasons (e.g. pregnancy).
- Age, occupation, health and personality of partner.

- Quality of relationship—threat of separation or divorce.
- Reaction of partner to patient's present illness.
- Communication, negotiation of differences, ability to confide, empathy.
- Dominance, submission, distance, trust, fidelity, jealousy.
- Problems, past and present, arguments, violence.
- Death of spouse? Separation (temporary or permanent) or divorce?
- Changes in sexual activities during relationship (e.g. ageing effects).
- Obstetric history: pregnancies, live births, terminations and miscarriages.

Children (present or earlier relationships): ages, sexes, names, present and past health, any psychiatric problems or treatment. Attitude towards children and future pregnancies. Proximity and contact with children not now living at home.

Assessing personality

Why assess personality?

Premorbid personality colours the presentation of mental illness. In addition, personality is one of the determinants of illness behaviour and adherence to treatment. The assessment of premorbid personality is, therefore, an essential part of a psychiatric assessment. In addition, personality disorders are common and burdensome conditions. Epidemiological research has shown that the prevalence of personality disorders increases steadily with each level of care: 10% in the community, 20% in primary care, and between 30 and 60% among samples of psychiatric patients as a main or ancillary diagnosis. People with a personality disorder have an increased risk of suicide, accidents, mental illness, and drug misuse, and they respond less well to treatment for mental illness. They are heavy users of health services and are, therefore, frequently encountered in clinical practice.

Definitions

Personality is a term used to describe enduring traits and behaviours that differentiate individuals from one another. Personality traits are usually present from adolescence, are stable over time, and are evident in a range of different environments. Personality disorders, on the other hand, are mental disorders characterized by enduring patterns of inner experience and behaviour that deviate from the individual's culture and are pervasive and inflexible. A core, defining feature of personality disorders is that the traits and associated behaviour are associated with significant personal, social, or occupational impairment. Features of the ICD-10 categories of personality disorder are given briefly below. The clinical assessment should aim to discover whether the features of one of these categories are present.

Categories or dimensions?

Doctors tend to prefer the use of categories when describing abnormal states. However, the categorical model of personality disturbance has its limitations. Criteria for categories of personality disorder frequently overlap and clinicians often disagree on whether categories are present or not. In fact, personality is probably more accurately conceptualized in terms of variation along at least five dimensions: (1) neuroticism, (2) extroversion, (3) openness to experience, (4) agreeableness, and (5) conscientiousness. Nevertheless, categories lead more readily to treatment decisions and convey more vividly the disturbance demonstrated by people with personality problems.

Use the term personality disorder cautiously!

People with personality disorders are often the most difficult people to be encountered in clinical practice. They do not readily reward staff and often intrude directly on their feelings. However, it is important to avoid using the term 'personality disorder' merely to explain disagreeable behaviour. There are stigmatizing effects of applying the label of personality disorder. Therefore, before the diagnosis is made, positive evidence must be sought.

Who should provide information?

Self-description is difficult and, in a clinical situation, the presence of mental illness may distort the assessment of personality. For these reasons, in addition to the patient's account of themselves, it is also desirable to obtain a corroborative account from an informant. The informant should be someone who has known the patient when they were free of symptoms for a number of years and preferably in more than one circumstance. The interview should enquire into positive as well as negative aspects of the patient's personality, as these may also guide the management strategy.

How should the interview proceed?

It is important to be sure that the informant or patient (as their own informant) understands that this interview concerns a time of life when the patient was well. Agree on that time (e.g. 5 years ago or before the marriage broke down) and focus the interview on that period. Begin by asking the informant an open-ended question, to describe in their own words how the patient was at that time. This response itself may indicate which diagnostic category of personality may be appropriate. However, if uninformative, the following more specific questions will probe for one of the ICD10 categories:

1. How does he/she get on with people?   (**paranoid**)
2. Would you describe him/her as a loner? (**schizoid**)
3. Does he/she trust other people?   (**paranoid, schizoid**)
4. What is his/her temper like?   (**dissocial**)

5. Is he/she impulsive?	**(emotionally unstable)**
6. Is he/she dramatic or irresponsible?	**(histrionic, dissocial)**
7. Is he/she a worrier or a shy person?	**(anxious)**
8. How much does he/she depend on others?	**(dependent)**
9. How does he/she respond to criticism?	**(anxious, paranoid)**
10. Does he/she have unusually high standards at work or home?	**(anankastic)**

Any one of these probes may point to one of the ICD-10 categories. The interviewer should, therefore, follow with subsidiary questions that concern the additional features of that category (see ICD-10 for details). In addition, the informant should be asked to indicate whether these features were generally present (e.g. not just at work) and whether the personality seemed responsible for personal suffering (e.g. periods of distress or unhappiness) or handicap in social or occupational life. From this information, abnormal premorbid personality may be identified or personality disorder diagnosed. If the patient is to be the informant, the same procedure can be followed. A number of reliable standardized assessment procedures for personality disorders now exist and, ideally, one of these should be used as part of the assessment. Examples of reliable assessment measures, developed in the UK for use in routine clinical settings, are the Standardized Assessment of Personality and the Personality Assessment Schedule.

Assessing family relationships

There are many reasons why it may be valuable to interview the family of the presenting patient (index patient), ranging from obtaining a good description of fits, seizures, and other altered states of consciousness to an examination of the family dynamics, for example to uncover possible maintaining influences in relation to the patient who relapses when a discharge date is decided. The index patient is, of course, included in the family meeting.

As a general rule, the earlier the family can be included in the investigation and treatment of a problem, the better—assuming the index patient is agreeable. It is important for the interviewer to be alert to the strengths and resources of the family, who will usually have tried hard to support and help their ill member before calling in the professionals. By the time they see you, they may be feeling demoralized and helpless. They may be angry with the patient and secretly blaming themselves or one another. Under these circumstances it is crucial that you do not add to their guilt or sense of failure.

How to manage a family interview

After initial introductions and an explanation of the setting (e.g. any one-way screen or closed-circuit television), start by thanking the family members for coming and acknowledging interruptions to school and work. Then state the purpose of the meeting by inviting them to help you help the index patient—as indeed they are experts by virtue of having known the person for longer and before he or she became ill. It is usually best to start by asking for a description of the problem, being sure to hear from each member of the family how they see it.

Even at this early stage, startlingly different descriptions of the problem are often given. It is valuable to define the problem as it affects the family now and to clarify that this may be different from how the problem began. The focus at this early stage in the interview is to translate the problem (described as an attribute of the index patient) into statements about relationships and differences in relationships among the family members. At all times it is important to note their non-verbal messages: posture, eye contact, interruptions, and emotional states (detachment, fear, sadness, etc.).

Current alliances in relation to the present problem may be asked about—who feels most upset by the problem, who notices first, who gets impatient first—obtaining a ranking of all members in relation to each question. It is very useful to track sequences of behaviour around the problem as this provides a detailed pattern of activity that is often stereotypic.

It is the family's attempt at a solution that has itself become part of the problem. By asking different family members for their explanation about how the pattern has evolved or why particular members take up particular roles in the sequence of behaviour, it is usually possible to uncover differences of opinion about what happens. It can be useful to ask what other approaches to the problem have been tried and why they were abandoned.

When you feel you have a clear picture of how the family tries and fails to help in relation to the immediate problem, it is time to enquire into how the problem affects other aspects of the family's life together. How does the family regroup when the index patient is ill, or away in hospital? Who takes over their tasks; who misses them most? By comparing and conducting current arrangements and role assignments with those before the problem began, certain hypotheses about what function the problem serves will emerge.

The final part of an initial family interview involves establishing with the family members whether or not they are willing to continue to work together with you in arriving at a better understanding of the problem and finding a way either of resolving it or of living with it. Alternatively you may discover there is such hostility towards the index patient or so much chaos, discord, or obstructiveness that it is clear the patient will have to be helped to live apart from the family. Although painful, this is usually much better accepted by the patient if the limits of what each family member is willing to offer in terms of help and support is made clear. For example, a couple who had divorced and both remarried, each had to say to their adult chronic schizophrenic daughter, in front of each other: 'You cannot, under any circumstances, live with me'. In this case the uncertainty had been perpetuated by each one saying: 'Wait until you are better, then you can live with me or possibly the other parent'.

There is so much information to take in, record, and interpret in a family interview that it is of great value to have a non-involved observer or a video recording. Any kind of electronic record requires the informed consent of the family at the beginning of the interview, with the option to delete the recording at the end.

Your observations may be recorded under the following headings.

1. Description of family members present
The family includes all those living in the same household, although children who have left home and relatives in other households who are significantly involved may be included.
- Note absent members.
- List names, ages, physical appearance, and mental state.

2. Description of problem
Use the words of family members. Include the problem as it began and the problem now. Record stereotypic pattern if elicited.

3. The stage of family life cycle
1. *Courtship*, marriage and the honeymoon period.
2. The *first child* alters the couple's view of themselves and each other as they make space for the baby.
3. *Subsequent children* each make demands for adjustment on existing family members.
4. The *children reach adolescence*, with the coming of puberty, sexual awakenings, and bids for independence, and face the challenge of leaving home.
5. The '*empty nest*', as the last child leaves home. The couple, having reached mid-life or later, face the dependence, illness, or death of their own parents, as well as what remains of their own life together.

Crises in families often arise when transition to the next stage is required, but for some reason cannot be negotiated successfully. Crises may result in a symptomatic member or marital difficulties, or both.

4. The genogram or family tree
This can be a powerful tool for eliciting trans-generational resonances. It is important to ask about stillbirths and other premature deaths; note the ages and date of death of grandparents, siblings, and children. Crises in the life cycles of the previous generation (the parents' families of origin) may illuminate difficulties in the presenting family. The occupation of each person should be indicated, if known.

5. The family structure

This refers to the existence of appropriate or inappropriate boundaries between different parts of the family: the boundary between the couple and each of their families of origin, as well as parents and children. Are there trans-generational alliances: father and daughter; mother and son; grandmother, mother, and daughter? Is one member of the family isolated (e.g. father) or scapegoated (e.g. a child who is different from the other siblings)? Facts informing these judgements can be elicited by asking about the routine daily activities: who does what with whom? How are mealtimes, bedtimes, housework, household chores, and leisure activities arranged? How is decision making done—do the couple consult one another? If not, who gets consulted and who does not? How are conflicts negotiated and resolved? Who has the final say? Who controls the finances? In families with an ill adolescent, the hierarchy is sometimes inverted: the parents are capriciously governed by their offspring.

6. Family roles and attitudes

In response to the questions above, it should also become clear whether particular family members are assigned by common agreement to certain roles, and how power, authority, and gender-specific activities are distributed. Implicit in these roles will be shared attitudes, although, when made explicit, differences of opinion may emerge. Acceptance of role assignment may be a way of avoiding conflict. Cultural and religious attitudes are often expressed in role assignments and expectations based on gender and birth order. A good way to find out more about cultural and religious views with which the interviewer is unfamiliar is to acknowledge difference and ignorance, and ask. This also allows the family members to describe how it is for them to belong to an ethnic minority and the impact of the dominant culture on their lives.

7. Communication and emotional climate

These aspects of the description of family relationships will first of all depend upon your observations of the family as they have responded to your questioning. Supplementary questioning can clarify how the various family members experience and think about one another. If, for example, a mother tends to answer for her daughter, the daughter can be asked, 'Does your mother always know what you are thinking?', or the father or other relative can be asked, 'How does your daughter manage to get her mother to speak for her?', or ask a sibling, 'Does your mother always speak for your sister or are there times when your sister can speak for herself?'.

Other common patterns are: one family member is frequently interrupted by another; one member is habitually silent and ignored, or disengaged or over-emotional; everyone talks at once; no one finishes a sentence; no one listens to anyone else; one member habitually defers to another.

There may be obvious omissions or evasions. Communication may be clear and direct or contradictory or obfuscating.

The emotional atmosphere may be free or frozen, cool and distant, or intensely over-involved. Dyads or subsystems may be locked in superiority and submission, condescension and self-effacement, cruelty and humiliation.

8. The hypothesis

This is an attempt to describe the problem in systemic terms: what maintains and prevents resolution of the problem in terms of the contribution made by each family member who, it is predicted, both gains and suffers from the status quo.

Assessing the social state

The social state provides a structure of five main headings, for each of which four main categories of information and assessment can be reported. In practice, the information may be written in columnar form or sequentially down the page. The four categories or columns will not all be needed if significant problems are absent. The format must allow for the possibility that only a very brief or highly distilled report will be required (or feasible) in some cases, while others may require a lot of detailed information. The social state refers to the patient's normal home setting (even if it is a doorway in the street) rather than the place in which the patient is examined. For a long-stay hospital patient, the usual home environment will initially be the ward. There are five main headings: accommodation, finances, home activities, outside activities, carers.

Accommodation

Under this heading the physical nature of the patient's residence and the identity of the people who normally provide the immediate social environment are described. The aim is to assess the type and quality of physical resources available to the patient in the home and to name the people who share the accommodation. Subheadings include:

- Type of accommodation.
- Physical amenities, personal space.
- Quality of accommodation.
- Identity of other people sharing the accommodation.
- Ease of access.
- Physical security.
- Nature and quality of neighbourhood.

Finances

This requires a description of the patient's financial status and use of welfare benefits, in order to assess income, monetary assets, liabilities, and capacity to handle money. Subheadings include:

- Sources of income (including welfare benefits).
- Capital.
- Expenditure (including special liabilities such as gambling).
- Debts (including threats of punitive action such as withdrawal of services or eviction).
- Budgeting capacity.

Home activities

The focus here is on daily events and activities within the home and the provision of both informal and professional support, and services from people visiting the home. Subheadings include:

- Way of spending a typical day (includes waking and rising, daily routines).
- Daily living skills (including personal hygiene, laundry, cooking, cleaning).
- Recreational activities.
- Visitors.
- Relationships with immediate neighbours.

Outside activities

The patient is seen in relationship to the local and wider community outside the home residence. Subheadings include:

- Occupation.
- Social contacts (family, friends, others).
- Shopping.
- Travel.
- Use of public amenities (e.g. pubs, cinema).
- Other outside leisure activities.
- Religious observance.
- Holidays.

Carers

Under this heading are listed the people who are individually identifiable as accepting a special responsibility for promoting and sustaining the patient's welfare. They may include family members, friends, other informal contacts, and members of professional agencies. Subheadings include:

Informal carers

- Caring relatives and friends.
- Relationships with other people within the home and local community.

- Attitudes to patient reported by others (or observed by assessor) within home.

Professional carers
- Staff members of NHS agencies (GP, psychiatric services, etc., and relationships with them).
- Staff members of other statutory agencies (social services, etc.).
- Members of voluntary bodies (including religious organizations).

Each of these headings is to be recorded using four vertical columns headed: Facts, Problems, Services, and Strengths:

1. *Facts*—aims to record the situation in terms of reported objective information from the patient or identified others (including the assessor).
2. *Problems*—comprises two kinds of element, which may be reported separately: subjective difficulties reported by the patient and objective difficulties observed by others.
3. *Services*—reports provisions already made at the time of assessment to alleviate some, but not necessarily all, of the problems identified. Inadequacies or overprovision may be commented on, but this area of the assessment report is not the place to record proposals about management.
4. *Strengths*—invites the assessor to report on positive features of the patient's social opportunities and functioning, which may serve to counterbalance the commonly prevailing negative tone of many psychiatric assessments by highlighting positive resources, relationships, and potentialities.

The social state should be inserted in the notes after the history and before the mental state examination. In this position it supplants and extends the information that may at present be recorded in the history, partly under 'previous personality' and partly under 'social history' or 'current circumstances'.

Cross-cultural assessments in psychiatry

Three elements of awareness, knowledge, and skill provide a sequence of cross-cultural training. The aim of such training is to provide the mental health professionals with an insight that increases the individual's control of assumptions that contribute to their behaviour, attitudes, and insight when dealing with patients from other cultures. The main goal of this section is to highlight some of the areas that may influence the psychiatrist's perceptions and stereotypes of individuals whose ethnic and racial background and cultural influences may be different from those of the psychiatrist. The doctor–patient interaction is affected by the training, past experience, social class, and ethnicity on the doctor's part and by the past experiences, educational and social background, and ethnicity of the patient. It is, of course, likely, that gender, socio-economic or educational status, lifestyle, job or professional role may overshadow the ethnic or racial identity of the patient. No culture is static, hence it is worth emphasizing that 'salient' culture for both the patient and the doctor will change from one situation to another.

If the cultural variables are over-emphasized, the provider is guilty of stereotyping the patient in one or two of the patient's identities, and if these are under-emphasized the doctor is guilty of insensitivity to the dynamic ranges of influences that may impinge on the interview. Mental health services are frequently looked down upon by members of minority ethnic groups because the institutions may be seen to replace support systems, may reflect Western dominant cultural values and implicit racism, may rely on psychological formulations that ignore cultural values and norms of ethnic minorities, and these institutions may be seen to be pandering to those who conform with the dominant culture.

Limitations of psychiatric assessments of cultural aspects

These limitations are linked with perceptions that suggest that all people's presentations to psychiatric services can be conceptualized and their distress fully understood by the mechanistic application of a standardized assessment interview. Duration, content, and focus of psychiatric assessment will depend greatly upon the purpose of the assessment—whether it is for diagnosis, management, rehabilitation, or psychotherapy. One of the commonest errors in cross-cultural assessments is to foreclose further or detailed enquiry as soon as the psychiatrist believes a clinical diagnosis has been reached, thereby completing the assessment.

It is better to use the assessment interviews as the basis for beginning to understand a patient's distress and to go on to develop a collaborative therapeutic relationship. The common reductionist approach emerges partly because of time restrictions, Western-style psychiatric training, necessity to act in an emergency, recognition that the communication is poor because of linguistic difficulties but also an uncertainty about the idioms of distress, and yet not having enough time to carry out a more thorough assessment. Some patients, irrespective of their ethnic status, will require a longer assessment before a comprehensive management plan can be formulated so that it truly reflects the *optional* package of interventions for that particular patient.

The inherent potential inadequacy of psychiatric assessment is amplified where the patient and the clinician come from different cultural backgrounds and the only common reference point is the culture of the clinic.

The optimal assessment requires special attention to several factors (Box 2.1).

Communication and cultural distance

The principles outlined here are not a recipe for 'how to do it' culture by culture, but are general guidelines aimed at ensuring safe and

Box 2.1 Special features of optimal cross-cultural psychiatric assessments

- Context of consultation—emergency or other; pathway into care.
- Patients' and their families' expectations of the consultation.
- Cultural patterns, taboos, physical distance, religious and other rites of passage.
- Potential for misinterpretation from both sides of consultation, especially racism, stereotyping, direct questioning, physical touch, distance, eye contact.
- Cultural as well as linguistic interpretation.
- Maximum pre-assessment information.
- Patients' and their families' explanations of causes, prognosis and treatment.
- Critical appraisal of missing information prior to completion of assessment.
- Assessment and appraisal contextualized by the culture and involvement of those properly familiar with the patient's culture and psychiatric nosology.

sensitive practice. *Before* commencing an assessment, it is important to find out about the culture and its essential features, including taboos, rites of passage, and religious values. The first and preferred language in which the patient communicates must be identified before commencing the interview. If this is not English, an appropriate interpreter must be identified who can also act as an adviser on non-verbal communication as well as identifying idioms of distress and 'emotional' words used by the patient.

The first step, therefore, must be an unstructured 10 minutes of 'emotional orientation', during which idioms of distress and emotional words can be identified that will give a clue towards the direction in which the assessment must proceed (see Box 2.2).

Essential historical data

Adverse events

Do not assume that the life events, adverse or otherwise, have the same significance for patients as they do for you or that they have only the significance described previously in the literature. Flexible enquiry will accurately elicit the impact of a patient's experiences. Similarly, admission or separation from children may be more traumatic than you might imagine, perhaps with culturally unacceptable implications.

Box 2.2   Setting up the assessment

- Know your limits—be aware of your own culture.
- Know your skills and be aware of how these can be blunted or affected by your culture.
- Know the patient's limits—assess predominant group within which the patient has status.
- Know the patient's skills and strengths.
- Know the family's limits—their language limitations, sense of urgency or crisis and realistic capacity of coping strategies available to them.
- Know the family's skills and strengths—do not denigrate these.
- Know the interpreter's role, skills, and limits. Meet with them before the assessment commences to identify their knowledge of culture and to identify sources of difference (e.g. dialect, tribe, religion, island).
- Agree on joint working—literal translation, cultural context of complaints, patients' and their families' objections to that particular interpreter.
- Confidentiality.

World view

This is the patient's perspective of the consultation and the emotional distress leading to this interaction. It has been described as the personal lens through which people differentially interpret events. This can be further divided into group and individual identity, and the patient's beliefs, values, and cognitive perceptions of the distress and the help being offered. This can be ascertained only after several semi-structured meetings with patients, family, advocates, religious and community spokesperson as nominated by the patient. This will give a profile of events, thought, and approaches to the problems of living deployed by the patient living in a majority culture that may be perceived as hostile. Such a collation of information will provide culturally contextualized, culturally sensitive information.

Acculturation

No culture remains static. With increasing contact with other cultures while living in close proximity to them along with globalization of cultures, the cultural expectation and behaviour will vary across generations. Acculturation must be seen as a multidimensional phenomenon that reflects the changes an individual goes through when exposed to a new culture. The concept of self varies across cultures, and changes brought about by cultures in individual self will vary across cultures. Acculturation is a feature for the individual, families,

Box 2.3 Assessment of migration

- How long ago did migration occur?
- Age of the patient at the time?
- Motives for migration (e.g. economic, political).
- Difficulties in migration?
- Reversibility of migration?
- Preparedness for migration.
- Differences between expectation and reality?
- Experiences before, during, and after arrival?
- Migrated alone or in a group?
- Initial intentions and expectations.
- Attitudes towards new country and culture.
- Helpfulness of the new society in adjustment.
- Previous similar experiences.

religious groups, and other culturally similar local groupings. It is not identical at each level and it is possible that degrees of acculturation will vary across different members of the family. Idioms of distress and expression of such distress along with help-seeking are all linked with processes of acculturation. Assess acculturation by determining the interval since migration and the reasons for migration (see Box 2.3) and by focusing on areas of religious activity, preferred dietary patterns, preferred leisure activities, and attitudes to traditional patterns of behaviour in the community (see Box 2.4).

Psychological/somatic mindedness

Often there is an assumption that a clear dichotomy exists between the psychological and somatic perceptions of distress. This is a false dichotomy and, furthermore, not a static one. The purpose for bearing this distinction in mind is to ascertain patients' ability to relate their symptoms in certain styles of communication, thereby allowing some help in treatment recommendations—whether physical or psychological therapies will be acceptable. Too often, the label of somatization is applied in a derogatory manner, especially if there is a poor communicative relationship. Although core depressive or psychotic symptoms are often regarded as universal, some see these constructs as disorders consistent with the developed world's conceptualization of distress and without universal applicability.

Previous experience of services and treatments

Such information is helpful in any psychiatric assessment; in working with patients from other cultures, previous bad experiences may deter the patient from using the services optimally. Previous experiences

---

Box 2.4   Assessment of acculturation: broad headings

• **Religion**	Practice
	Frequency
	Who attends? Where?
• **Languages**	Spoken
	Where?
	Frequency?
• **Marriage/Family**	Type
	Attitudes to marriage
	Responsibility at home? Gender roles?
	Arranged marriages?
• **Employment**	Working with others of same ethnicity?
	Relationship?
	Work ethic?
• **Leisure activities**	What interests?
	Languages spoken
	Films? Music? Preference.
• **Food**	Type; shopping, where?
• **Aspirations and attitudes to self**	

---

may not necessarily have occurred in this country and the criteria for help-seeking and service provision may differ widely, thereby making acceptability of statutory services problematic.

Racism

Members from ethnic minorities are likely to have experienced discrimination in one or more fields of daily activities (e.g., legal, financial, educational, or healthcare activities). This may be full-blown open discriminatory experience or suspected prejudicial treatment. This discriminatory behaviour could be on account of skin colour, religion, language, sex, race, or other factors that may well be masked under a broader umbrella. Do not underestimate the impact of such events and do not assume that you understand the context. Ask about such events in a careful, paced, sensitive manner so that the patient may respond accordingly. Even if perceived racist experiences do not contribute directly to the patient's presentation, treat such reports with respect and do not dismiss them as unimportant or irrelevant. If a patient finds that such experiences are not being understood or taken seriously, they may find it difficult to trust you with more sensitive information. Your attempts to focus away from these experiences on to only psychiatrically relevant issues will be sensed and interpreted as evidence of further power imbalance, and could fracture a budding treatment alliance. Anyone who has been exposed to these experiences directly or indirectly is understandably sensitive to repeated trauma of this kind and may interpret an unsatisfactory assessment and consultation as discriminatory.

Limitations of the standard mental state examination (MSE)

The MSE must be thorough and detailed, as with any other patient. However, where the patient does not share the mental health professional's culture (regardless of skin colour) then any symptoms and signs must be appraised critically in a cultural context and the appraisal revisited in response to emergence of more information. Various cultural, religious, and social groups are more likely to have varying and possibly unique idioms of distress, but to list them would suggest that clinicians could and should follow a recipe of cultural assessment based on the initial—and perhaps erroneous—impressions regarding the impact of cultural, religious, and social differences. However, application of diagnostic processes without due attention to socio-cultural influences (and cultural context) is likely to meet with numerous pitfalls.

Behaviour

Behaviours that, to the assessing clinician, may appear odd or bizarre may have a culturally sanctioned role. For example, speaking in tongues, excessive religiosity, and trance possession are culturally sanctioned. These phenomena can be evaluated only by carefully recording the behaviour, the patient's explanation for it, and the family and the cultural group's response to it. These views, if a sign of illness, may change as the patient recovers, and become important signs by which the patients, their carers, and others in the folk sector may in the future identify a relapse. Unusual behaviour that is not clearly understandable is too readily assigned as evidence of psychosis without due attention to the adaptive or coping potential of the behaviour.

Aggression

Aggression is often labelled as being a manifestation of psychosis. Potential aggression is especially difficult to anticipate and the interviewer may err on the side of caution by intervening too early if feeling threatened. Early intervention may well jeopardize any future treatment alliance. 'Our biology interacts with culturally shaped experiences to produce frustration and then to assert dominance and respond in a variety of ways, of which aggression is one.' The only way to assess a potentially aggressive patient is to have no doubt about your safety. Ensure that you are accompanied and encourage a relative or friend of the patient to join you (see p. 19). There may be cultural norms of frustration, conflict resolution, and aggression sanctions. Do not be prompted to anticipate an aggressive situation through your own fear of assault and uncertainty about a patient with whom you do not share cultural values, norms, and mores.

Hallucinations

Check exact experiences, consistency, and especially differentiate from illusions and suggestibility states. If the patient uses figures of speech inexactly to articulate their illness experience, the clinician must avoid erroneously identifying them as hallucinations. It has been demonstrated that among their black sample with bipolar affective illness, 85% had a previous diagnosis of schizophrenia and a higher than expected proportion had auditory hallucinations. The presence of visual phenomena is especially difficult to locate firmly within the standard psychopathology framework.

Delusions

The traditional definition of delusion does take the role of culture and its context into account. There is, of course, a hypothetical possibility that if the examiner is not clear about the cultural values a delusional experience may be misattributed. Religious ideas, culturally sanctioned explanations, spiritual or cosmic explanations must be carefully identified and documented verbatim. Do not just record your impressions. Always consider alternative reasons for a patient's beliefs with their relatives or advocates. Again, record intact their responses. If a belief is culturally unfamiliar and is coupled with functional impairment or culturally inappropriate (with their culture) behaviour then it is likely to be a sign of illness.

First-rank symptoms

World Health Organization studies have demonstrated the existence of core symptoms of schizophrenia across cultures. There is still debate in some anthropological quarters about the suitability and validity of such studies. There is considerable concern that first-rank symptoms can occur in other psychiatric states and also in the course of culturally sanctioned methods of resolving distress (e.g. passivity, possession, exorcism, delusions of control). Anecdotal evidence also suggests that some of the first-rank symptoms are best picked up if a patient's first or preferred language is used for interviewing.

Cognitive assessment

The standard cognitive assessment may yield very little diagnostic psychopathology if used blindly across cultures, especially with different languages. It is better to obtain third-party information on the memory failure and intellectual decline. If schedules of cognitive assessment are available in the patient's primary language these must be employed, bearing in mind the patient's level of education; once again, the help of an advocate or a team member who speaks the patient's first language can be invaluable.

Management of patients from other cultures

The management of patients from other cultures must be balanced with the patient's wishes, taking account of cultural distance and that you may be making a clinical decision on the basis of information that may be less than adequate. Therefore, a careful risk assessment is warranted. Do not prescribe symptomatically if the diagnosis remains unclear. This will lead to false expectations on the part of the patient and may expose them to adverse side-effects which render them less inclined to return or take medication in the future.

If the problem is not urgent and there is sufficient time, arrange for a further assessment. This will allow you to think about the patient's presentation, receive supervision, and obtain corroborative information from past records, other health professionals, family members, etc., and it will also give you a further opportunity of garnering information on the patient's culture. Do let the patient know that you will be doing this.

Inferences

Be sure to discuss you inferences, diagnosis, and management plans with the patient and his or her advocates or identified family members. The appropriateness of aetiological and diagnostic inferences should be considered with an awareness that such a process and the rules thereof are influenced by culture. Your assumptions about these inferences should be checked with the patient. If the patient and other interested parties, including advocates, disagree with your intended management plan, arrange to meet and discuss risk assessment. You should not alienate valuable community support, or your aftercare plans may be compromised or the community team may end up carrying a bigger level of involvement than is possible.

Consultation dynamics

As discussed above, the patient's models of what the doctor does may be quite different from what you are able to offer. Some people from minority ethnic groups will have a great respect for health professionals—the doctor in particular—such that they may not confront, question, disagree, or point out the problems they may be facing. Although not a crisis, such a problem may manifest later as selective omission of medication, inaccurate reporting of symptoms, or consultation with other healers, who may prove to be beneficial in treatment of illness although others may deter the patient from attending services or, more commonly, offer excessive reassurance or promise of miraculous cure which will encourage the patient to disengage with the statutory sector.

Box 2.5 Good practice points

- For each party involved in the consultation, elicit the first language, religion, self-defined ethnicity, identification with specific cultural groups.
- Define and redefine terms used by you and the patient to ensure shared understanding of problems.
- Identify emotional idioms of distress and develop a shared vocabulary with the patient.
- Ask for clarification if symptoms or signs appear unusual or unfamiliar.
- Assume nothing about the patient. Do not be judgmental about patterns of communication or domination of the clinical interview by one family member—this may be cultural or the family's style of communication.
- Be sensitive to the effects of your action, the setting, or the referral mode that jeopardizes trust. Communicate total confidentiality. Identify the scenario where the patient may be most comfortable and relaxed (e.g. with family, alone).
- Be sensitive to religious and social taboos.
- Do not ask children to interpret. Avoid relatives interpreting unless an emergency and delay will be detrimental to the patient.
- Involve patient advocates early, with the patient's consent.
- Discuss the findings with an independent person properly familiar with the culture, within the bounds of strict confidentiality.

The psychiatric interview with children

Some differences from interviewing adults

1. The child is *brought*—the reasons may not have been explained or they may be inaccurate. The child may believe he or she is going to be told off, taken away, kept, or hurt. They may be waiting for a blood test or operation.

2. The child is not the main informant.

3. The child may not answer any questions at all, no matter how experienced the psychiatrist. Sometimes children or even teenagers who will not speak can be persuaded to draw or play a game.

4. The experience of *uninterrupted* time with total attention from a sympathetic adult will be new to many children.

Setting

There are great advantages in ensuring that diagnostic interviews with children of similar age are broadly comparable. The interview room should be arranged so that only the objects that the psychiatrist considers will be needed are in view. The toys and games that are available need to be chosen with care so as to facilitate the types of observations that are of greatest diagnostic value. Observation of a child is much more difficult in a room cluttered with toys. For the child aged 6 years or more it is usually preferable to spend most of the interview talking with the child in the manner outlined below. With younger children and those with language or global delay there will need to be a greater reliance on non-verbal communication, and interaction will generally be easier if it occurs in a play situation.

With more mature children or adolescents, the interview may often take more of the form of the adult psychiatric interview, but considerable modifications are still required because adults often come to the clinic because of their own concern over their problems. By contrast, the child or adolescent is generally referred because of someone else's concern.

General advice

- Be non-judgemental.
- Be prepared to specify limits—destruction and rage are not cathartic. 'That's not what people do here', 'I want you to stop doing that.'
- Avoid long silences which can become persecutory, particularly for adolescents—some can be engaged in a game, some will respond to 'I wonder whether…'
- Accept pictures if offered, and keep them safely, because they will be asked about another time. Pictures should not be put in the place of honour on the wall: it will not be possible to do this for all the children who come and someone else may take them down.
- Do not speak in an artificial voice—children are quite tone responsive.
- Do not rush in with direct interpretations.
- Do not let the child take toys out of the room. 'Sorry, these toys belong to the hospital and there would be none for you to play with if you took one home every time.'
- Warn about the end of the session 5 minutes before it finishes.

Common errors

- To keep off relevant, but difficult, topics in pursuit of a pleasant experience for the child.
- To side with the child instead of displaying a constructive neutrality.
- To lead a suggestible child into inappropriate answers.
- To build castles in the air on the nods of mute children.

Engagement

A short diagnostic family interview (10–15 minutes' duration) provides a useful initial contact with the family. This can be followed by more formal history taking, an individual interview with the child, and psychometric assessment as necessary. The clinician begins by explaining who he or she is (for example, in the case of young children: 'I am a doctor who helps children and families with their problems and muddles') and the planned structure of the assessment. The family can then be asked to introduce themselves. Subsequently, it is helpful to ask the parent/carers whether it would be alright to talk to the children first, and to engage the children individually on such (potentially) neutral topics as where they go to school and what that is like, whether they have friends, the names of their friends, what they like doing when at home or with friends, what they are good at. Having tried to engage all the children briefly in this way, it is important to explore with them why they think their parents decided that they should attend, preferably directing the question to a sibling of the referred child rather than to that child himself or herself. The children are then encouraged to check with their parent(s) whether their understanding regarding the reason for the appointment is correct. Exploration with the children regarding reason for referral facilitates family communication around this issue, while at the same time clarifying the reasons for referral.

This joint time allows for the beginnings of an engagement with the children and family while observing family communication patterns, the emotional tone employed during communication (warm, critical, hostile, detached, understanding), and alliances between family members. Parents are generally pleased that time has been spent engaging their children in conversation, and this time may act as a useful model for parents who have difficulty communicating with their child(ren).

Subsequent to the family interview, if co-workers are available it is useful to split up so that one person can elicit a more formal history from the parents, while another can engage the child in an individual interview or more formal assessment. If siblings are present, they may be supervised by child-care staff (if available at the clinic), by an accompanying relative or family friend, or a parent may decide to monitor them while the other parent continues to participate in the assessment process. Information about the parent–child relationship can be gleaned from the parent's handling of the separation from the child and the child's response.

Children aged at least 6 years

Children will often be on the defensive, knowing that complaints have been made to the doctor about their behaviour. It is, therefore, usually unwise to make any mention of the complaints at the beginning of the interview. The doctor should make it clear by their behaviour towards the children that they are not acting as a judge or as someone who is going to correct or criticize. The aim is rather to show respect for the children as individuals and interest in what they say and do.

If children are expected to sit down for part of the interview, restless or uninhibited behaviour will be more readily observed. The first aim is to get them relaxed and talking freely, to assess the relationship they are able to form in such a setting, the level and lability of their mood, their conversation, and any habitual mannerisms. In order to provide an adequate sample of behaviour, there should be about 15 minutes of unstructured conversation. The children should be encouraged to talk about recent events and activities, what sort of things they like doing after school and at weekends, what they do with their friends and families, the names of their friends, the games they play, what they enjoy and do not enjoy at school, etc. They may also be asked about their hopes for the future, and what they want to do when they leave school or are grown up.

Respond with interest, concern, or enthusiasm as may be appropriate (to set a relaxed and informal atmosphere, to try to elicit a range of emotions, and to assess the emotional responsiveness of the child and the kind of relationship they form with the examiner). The interview must be geared to the child's age, intelligence, and interests. If the emotional responsiveness of the child is to be adequately assessed, it is necessary for the psychiatrist also to show a range of emotions (being more serious or concerned when asking about feelings of distress or worry, and more lively when responding to children's accounts of what interests or amuses them). Emotionally loaded topics should be pursued as they arise. The examiner's response should not block or lead away from expression of pathology or discomfort.

The children should then be questioned sympathetically about the specific information that is to be elicited. Open questions are usually preferable and multiple choice questions are sometimes useful. Specific examples of relevant feelings or events should be asked for. Indirect statements—'I knew a boy once about your age who…'—may be productive. (If the child accepts this convention there is no need to challenge it with statements such as, 'This boy is you, isn't it?')

It is expedient to ease off topics that seem too threatening, but the interviewer should return to them. Does the child ever feel lonely, get into fights, get teased, or picked on? Are they picked on more than most other children? Why do they think they are picked on? Similarly, they should be asked how they get on with their brothers and sisters. If they get into fights, do they like fighting, are they 'real' fights or 'friendly' fights?

The children should be asked specifically about worries, ruminations, fears, unhappiness, bad dreams, and the sort of things that make them feel angry. For example, they might be asked, 'Most people tend to worry about some things. What kind of things do you worry about? Do you ever lie awake at night worrying about things? Do you ever get nasty thoughts on your mind that you cannot get rid of? Do you ever get fed up? Miserable? Cry? Feel really unhappy?' Suicidal thoughts should be pursued where appropriate. 'Are there things you are particularly afraid of? What about the dark? Spiders? Dogs? Monsters? Do you ever dream? What about bad dreams? Or nightmares? What kind of things make you angry and annoyed?'

If anything positive should come up in answer to these questions, the psychiatrist should probe regarding the severity, frequency, and setting of the emotions (e.g. 'Do you ever feel so miserable that you want to go away and hide? Or that you want to run away? When was the last time that happened? How often do you feel like that? What sort of things make you fed up? Do you feel like that at home? … at school, etc.').

Children can be very suggestible and will sometimes produce the answers that they think the doctor wants. However, the anxious or depressed child can usually be distinguished by the affective state when talking about worries, fears, feeling fed-up, etc. Although it is important to ask the child systematically about these issues, it is also necessary for much of the interview to consist of neutral or cheerful topics. Note whether the child mentions worries spontaneously or extends answers on those topics beyond the questions.

The child should be asked to draw a picture of someone or of a house and everyone who lives in it, and encouraged to talk about it. This provides the opportunity to assess their natural skills, persistence, and distractibility, and also their attitudes and feelings, in so far as they are expressed in the drawing and what they say about the drawing. Handedness and fine motor skills can be assessed at the same time.

To assess attention span, persistence, and distractibility; children should be given some tasks within their ability, but near to its limits. The drawing constitutes one task; in addition they might be asked to give days of the week forwards and backwards, the months of the year, and also do some simple arithmetic (such as serial 7s from 100, serial 3s from 30, addition, subtraction, or multiplication tables). This is one situation in the interview where the child is stressed; emotionally loaded discussion is another. Tics and involuntary movements are often at their most apparent when the child is under stress, and should also be noted throughout the interview.

Note that *tics* are rapid, stereotyped, repetitive, non-rhythmic, predictable, purposeless contractions of functionally related muscle groups, which can usually be imitated or suppressed voluntarily for a time; *stereotypies* are voluntary, repeated, isolated, identical, predictable, often rhythmic actions, in which whole areas of the body are involved; *mannerisms* are odd, stylized embellishments of goal-directed movement. Notice also whether the level of activity is increased: *restlessness* is an inability to remain in seat appropriately, whereas *fidgetiness* refers to squirming in the seat, or movements of parts of the body but not the whole child.

Children aged below 6 years

A play setting is usually more appropriate for a child of 6 years or less; depending on the maturity of the child, it may sometimes be desirable to use a play-interview with older children.

Games and toys should be chosen to: (1) be suitable for the child's age, gender, and social background; (2) provide an interaction with the interviewer; and (3) encourage communication and imaginative play. The psychiatrist should get used to using a small range of toys, for example farm animals, colours, a doll's house with figures, plasticine. Board games such as chess are not very productive. Imaginative games such as the squiggle game (making a drawing out of the child's squiggle and getting the child to do the same out of your squiggle), playing with family figures, etc. may offer the best opportunity for eliciting a range of behaviour and emotions. Where possible, the child should be seen without the parents. However, with very young children it may often be better to allow the mother to come in with the child first and then, after a short while, she can withdraw from the situation or leave the room.

It is important to allow the child to get used to the situation before the examiner makes an approach. Initially, it may be useful simply to let the child explore the room and the toys while the doctor makes a friendly remark or two, and responds to the child's approaches, but makes no approach directly. The speed with which the child may be engaged in interaction and the way in which the approach is best made will vary considerably and must be judged in relation to each individual child. An attempt should be made to provide some activity known to interest the child.

The play situation should be utilized to make the same kind of assessment with the older child and, where appropriate, the child should be questioned in a manner suitable for their level of maturity. Young children cannot be expected to give descriptions of how they feel or to answer complex questions with long words about abstract concepts. Nevertheless, many can explain what they do at home, whom they play with, etc.

Scheme for description of mental state

General description

Appearance, attractiveness, manner, style of dress, any evidence of neglect; response to separation from parents, entering the interview room and the doctor's attempts to make contact.

Child's adjustment to the situation

Apprehension, appropriate or excessive reserve, emerging confidence, friendliness, disruption, and age appropriateness. Topics of spontaneous conversation.

Motor activity

1. Amount of movement—reduced or increased.
2. Coordination.
3. Involuntary movements.
4. Posturing.
5. Rituals.
6. Hyperventilation.

If any problems are noted, fuller neurological evaluation is needed.

Language

1. Hearing: sounds, speech.
2. Comprehension.
3. Speech, vocalization, babble:
   (a) spontaneity
   (b) quantity, rate and rhythm (e.g. stuttering)
   (c) pattern of intonation and stress
   (d) articulation (e.g. dysarthria)
   (e) grammatical accuracy and complexity
   (f) specific abnormalities (e.g. echoing, stereotyped features, I/you reversals (with written example if appropriate).
4. Gesture: imitation, comprehension, use.

If any problems are noted, go to p. 52.

Social response to interviewer

1. Social responsiveness to examiner's manner and comments (e.g. praise, reward).
2. Rapport and eye contact: quality, quantity.
3. Reciprocity and empathy.
4. Social style (e.g. reserved, shy, expansive).
5. Disinhibited, cheeky, precocious, teasing.
6. Negativistic, non-compliant, untruthful, surly.
7. Ingratiating, manipulative.

If any problems are noted, go to pp. 49–50.

Affect

1. Emotional expressiveness and range.
2. Happiness.
3. Anxiety: free-floating, situational, or specific phobias.
4. Panic attacks.

5. Observable tension.
6. Signs of autonomic disturbance.
7. Tearfulness.
8. Sadness, wretchedness, despair, apathy.
9. Thoughts of suicide or running away.
10. Shame, embarrassment, perplexity.
11. Anger, aggressiveness.
12. Irritability.

Thought content

1. Worries, fears.
2. Preoccupations, obsessions, suspicions.
3. Hopelessness, guilt.
4. Low self-esteem, self-hatred.
5. Fantasies or wishes:
   (a) spontaneously mentioned
   (b) evoked (e.g. three wishes).
6. Quality of ideation/play.
7. Abnormal beliefs or experiences.

Cognition

1. Attention span, distractibility.
2. Persistence.
3. Curiosity.
4. Orientation in time and space.
5. Memory.

Attainment

Reading, spelling, and arithmetic are best assessed with standardized tests (e.g. Neale and Schonell for reading). If a formal assessment by a psychologist is not available, the child should be asked to read simple passages, to recall their gist, and to write a sentence about a previous event. The fluency, accuracy, and comprehension of reading are all important. This testing is even more necessary for children with disturbed behaviour or frustration in the classroom.

Standardized measures

An increasing number of rating scales for parents and teachers is available, and standardized structured or semi-structured interviews are used for some clinical purposes.

Advantages of explicit and formalized interviewing schemes are that they ensure systematic cover of key parts, and can provide standards of whether a problem is severe enough to be deviant. A corresponding disadvantage is that they cannot cover everything. The crucial aspect of an individual case may be uncommon or even unique. Standardized schemes may divert attention away from the individually significant to what is common. They need to be supplemented with the general clinical enquiry that is described here. Most symptoms in child psychiatry are on a continuum with normality. The judgement of what constitutes a disorder should be based not only on the levels of symptoms, but also on an assessment of their impact on child and family.

Rating scales for parents and teachers are valuable as group tests, and sometimes for screening purposes. However, they are not yet sufficiently sensitive or specific for diagnosing an individual child. Rater effects, as well as the child's behaviour, will determine how they are completed.

Interviewer's subjective response to child

A brief sentence is sufficient.

Conclusion

Finally, an opinion should be expressed on whether (and how) the child's mental state departs from that expected in relation to age, IQ, sex, and social background.

Sources of information

Children are usually referred as a result of adult concern about their behaviour. Much more reliance is placed on accounts derived from a variety of informants than is usual in adult psychiatry. Accounts are needed of the child's behaviour and emotions at home, at school or playgroup, and as observed during the assessment.

The child is developing continuously. Symptoms and behavioural problems change with developmental stages, as do emotional needs. Even more than with adults, the assessment of behaviour and mental state needs to focus on the aspects relevant to the individual child's developmental stage.

Children's social and personal development is strongly influenced by the relationships formed at home and at school. The attitudes of, and the quality of relationships with, adult care-givers need assessment as well as the child's development.

Interviewing parents

The history taking consists of two aspects: (1) obtaining information about events and behaviour; and (2) recording expressed feelings, emotions, or attitudes concerning these events or the individuals participating in them. Because much of the interview is concerned with eliciting precise factual material, it is important to establish early that the interviewer is interested in feelings as well as events.

Care should be taken to encourage positive and negative attitudes to an equal extent. Where the informant's feelings are in doubt, questions such as 'Does this kind of thing ever cause an atmosphere in the home?' or 'Does that ever make you feel on edge?' are also useful, but should be used sparingly. In assessing the informant's feelings and emotions, attention should be paid to the way things are said as well as to what is said. Differences in the tone of voice, shown in the speed, pitch, and intensity of speech, can be important in the recognition of emotions. Particular attention should be paid to expressed criticism, hostility, and warmth, and to whom it is directed. Facial expressions and gestures should also be taken into account.

It is desirable, when possible, to see both the mother and the father. The child's relationship with father is as important as that with mother, although its importance will be for somewhat different aspects of development. It is undesirable to have to rely only on a second-hand account of the father obtained from the mother. An interview with two parents together will often provide a good opportunity of observing parental interaction and relationships. If the parents are divorced or separated and the child spends time with each of them, it may be more appropriate to see the other parent on a separate occasion, as well as seeing any new, significant adults in the family.

Present complaint

The interview with the parents begins with an enquiry about the problems or difficulties that are the chief cause of concern to the informant. The parents should tell their story in their own words and then be asked whether there are any other difficulties. *Recent examples* of the problems should always be obtained as well as the *frequency* of the behaviour, the *severity*, and the *context* of its occurrence (e.g. at school or when the child is away from home). The circumstances that *antecede or precipitate* the behaviour and those that *ameliorate or aggravate* the difficulties should always be noted. Determine the time of onset of the difficulties and go back to the point in the child's development when behaviour or emotions first appeared unusual, abnormal, or a cause for concern. Were there stresses at that time?

This part of the interview provides a good opportunity to assess parental feelings, attitudes, and beliefs about the problem, and these should be described carefully. In addition, the interviewer should find out what strategies have been used to deal with the problem, and how much success or failure has been experienced with each method. It is useful, too, at this point to find out what effect the symptom has had on the rest of the family. If appropriate, the interviewer should also enquire what led to the seeking of help with regard to the child's problem and why help has been sought now rather than at any other time.

If delayed or deviant development is prominent, whether global or specific, turn to pp. 55–9. The assessment of children with developmental disorders.

Systematic questioning

Review of other symptoms

Emotions Is the child happy or miserable? What makes them cry? Are they worried, depressed, suicidal, irritable, sulky? Do they show temper? Exhibit fears and panics? Are there tears on getting to school, or even school refusal? Are they fussy? Are there specific things or situations that arouse fear? Are there any compulsions to do things? (NB: Obsessions and compulsions in children are not necessarily accompanied by a subjective sense of resistance and may present as a handicapping ritual that cannot be explained.)

Antisocial trends Is the child disobedient? Destructive? Do they set fires? Tell lies? Steal? Are these problems only at home, or outside? Do they happen when solitary or with others? How are the problems dealt with? Has there been truanting or running away? Do they smoke, drink, sniff glue, or take drugs? Are they cruel to animals? Has there been any trouble with the police? *If yes to any of these, obtain details and enquire about the child's attitudes to discipline.*

Activity and concentration Is the child overactive or restless? Will they stay still if expected to, or are they always fidgety? How good is their concentration and what is the longest time they can concentrate on something interesting? Is there any change or loss of interest?

Eating, sleeping, and elimination Are there eating difficulties at home or at school? Do they show food refusal or faddiness? Pica? Do they have sleeping difficulties—poor settling at night, waking in the night, nightmares? What are the sleeping arrangements? Is there enuresis—diurnal or nocturnal? Wetting when away from home? Have they ever been dry? Is there soiling or smearing? Have they ever been clean? Where is the lavatory? (Regularity of function is also a temperamental attribute.)

Current functioning

Typical day A time budget helps to establish the context for children who are being assessed. In term time, who wakes up first? What happens? Who gets breakfast? How do the children behave first thing? How long do they take to get dressed? Who takes them to school? What are they like when they get home? What do they do then? How closely are they supervised? How do they behave during the evening meal; and when they are going to bed? What are the activities, and who provides care, during the school holidays? (NB: This enquiry is essentially to establish the framework; do not spend a long time on meticulous recording of exact details.)

Peer relationships Although poor peer relationships are not a specific disorder, they are a good indicator of general adjustment. What are the names of any friends? What do they do together? How close are they, how long have they been friends, do they visit each other's houses? Do other children reject or ignore? Does the child seek social contact or prefer to be solitary? Are peer relationships only with a deviant group?

Sibling relationships How do they get on? Is the child particularly attached to any siblings? How is this shown? Are there squabbles and with whom? Do they come to blows? Is there jealousy?

Relationships with adults (This is also a convenient time to discover parental attitudes.) How does the child get on with mother/father? How is affection shown? Are they an easy child to get on with? How do they compare with other children? Whom do they take after and how? How do they get on with other adults? With teachers? Is there anyone to whom they are particularly attached? Does anyone help to look after them? What is it about them that parents find hardest to tolerate?

Family history and circumstances

Family structure, family life, and relationships
Take note of the appearance, manner, and mental state of parental informant(s).

Persons in home Obtain a list. It may be helpful to draw a family tree. Ask about the age, religion, occupation, education, and health of each person. Have the child's parents been married before? Are they adopted or fostered? Mother's pregnancies, including miscarriages and stillbirths. Make sure biological parents are identified. Obtain the same details about a parent or siblings who live away from home.

Important people outside the home For example, for grandparents and parental sibs, establish what contact there is and the child's relationship. Obtain a sketch of the parent's own childhood.

Parental relationship How do the parents get on with each other? What things do they enjoy doing together? How do they spend evenings and weekends? To what extent does the father participate in child care, discipline, and household tasks?

Parental–Child interaction What activities are done by parent and child jointly? Do they go out together? Play together? Help with homework? Help make things?

Child's participation in family activities Does the child help with dressing, feeding, etc? Who helps? Does the child help with washing up, shopping, errands, etc?

Family patterns of relationships Are they the mother's child or father's child? Do they confide in father or in mother? What attachments to other adults are there?

Rules at home Do they have bedtime rules? Do they climb on furniture? Leave the house without saying where they're going, etc? Are there restrictions on friends, staying out late, reading or TV? Who monitors the child's behaviour? Who reprimands? What method of punishment is used? Do they have pocket money?

Family history of medical and mental health problems
A history of disorders in biological relatives needs to be taken carefully because of the importance of genetic factors. For each first-degree relative, question should be asked to determine the presence or absence of any psychiatric disorders, psychiatric treatment, depression, suicide, language delay, difficulty learning to read, enuresis, social oddness, alcoholism, epilepsy, court appearances. Age of onset is helpful. For the more extended family, establish not only which members of the family, if any, have had mental problems but their exact position in the family, and the other members who have not had problems. The pattern of transmission, if there is a familial disorder, needs to be established.

Home circumstances
A home visit is not done routinely, but when indicated it provides the best quality information and can often throw light on puzzling aspects of the history. Does the child live in a house or flat? How many rooms are there? Are there others in the home? What are the sleeping arrangements? Facilities (bath, lavatory, etc.)?

Other care arrangements Does anyone else look after them—grandparents, baby minder, neighbour after school, au pair, divorced parent at weekends, etc.?

Finances What sources of finance are there? Are there any difficulties?

Neighbourhood How long has the child lived there? Give a description of the area. Is it liked or disliked? Is there conflict with their neighbours? Is there any environmental threat (e.g. frequent assaults)?

Personal history

A general account of the art of eliciting a developmental history is to be found on pp. 55–8, on the assessment of children with developmental disorders.

Pregnancy Was it planned or not, and in what circumstances? (e.g. adverse reaction of mother's own parents, abandoned by baby's father). Were there complications such as toxaemia or haemorrhage, or stresses such as infection, smoking, alcohol, drugs, or X-rays?

Delivery Enquire about the place of birth (home or hospital), length of labour, presentation, mode of delivery, maturity, birth-weight, complications? Was resuscitation given—incubator or special care baby unit? Give details of the mother's health during and after pregnancy, including depression.

Neonatal period Were there difficulties breathing or sucking? Cyanotic attacks? Convulsions? Jaundice? Floppiness? Infection? Were they kept in hospital longer than usual?

Feeding and sleep pattern in infancy Were they breast-fed or bottle-fed? When were they weaned? Were there difficulties? Normal sleep pattern? Describe any difficulties.

Social development in infancy Were they placid or active? Irritable? What was their response to mother? Did they cry a lot? What other attachments did they have?

Milestones Useful stages to ask about: sitting unsupported, walking unaided, first word with meaning, and first two-word phrases. Comparison with siblings' development is helpful when exact stages are not remembered. Currently, do they speak as well as others of the same age, or do they have difficulty in understanding or producing speech, or in pronunciation, such as a lisp, baby talk or stutter? *If marked difficulties, turn to Table 3.1.* Do they show clumsiness? Is there preference for a particular hand and foot? Do they have any twitches? Where? Head banging? Habits or rituals?

Bladder and bowel control When were they dry by day and by night? (This is expected by the age of 5 years.) When did they have bowel control? (This is expected by the age of 4 years.) Were there any difficulties? Was training used? If so, how was it done? Who trained: childminders, nurseries, playgroups? How did the child respond?

Illness and allergies Were they ever in hospital—inpatient, outpatient, clinic, operations, accidents? Have they had any serious illnesses—measles, meningitis, encephalitis, fits, or convulsions? Are they off school at all? Do they suffer from asthma, headaches, stomach aches, or bilious attacks? How good is their sight and hearing? Do they suffer from fainting, fits, or absences? Any evidence of abnormal reactions to drugs or particular foods?

Separations Have they ever been away from home without their parents or been separated while in hospital? Have they been apart from their parents for as long as 4 weeks? How were they looked after? What were the circumstances? How did they react?

Failures of care Has there been any serious adversity in the past? Has caring been inadequate at any point (e.g. through illness incapacity or absence of a parent)? Has the child ever been maltreated (e.g. by physical or sexual abuse)?

Table 3.1 Scheme for current speech and language

1. *Limitation*—of housework, etc.

2. *Inner language*—meaningful use of miniature objects, pretend play, drawing

3. *Comprehension of gesture*

4. *Comprehension of spoken language*
   Hearing: response to sounds; response to being called by name; reaction to loud noises; reaction to quiet, meaningful sounds (mother's footsteps, noise of spoon in dish, food being prepared, door opening, rattle, etc.); ever thought deaf?
   Listening and attention
   Understanding: response to simple and complicated instructions with and without gesture (get details of examples)

5. *Vocalization and babble (non-speaking child)*
   Amount
   Complexity
   Quality
   Social usage—does the child babble back to you?

6. *Language production*
   Mode: gesture, pointing; taking by hand; speech
   Complexity: syntactical and semantic; length of sentences; vocabulary; use of personal pronouns, etc.
   Qualities: echoing, stereotyped features, I/you confusion, made up words, other oddities
   Amount
   Use of social communication: asking for things; to comment or chat to and fro; in reply to questions; mute in certain situations

7. *Word–sound production*
   Any difficulties in pronunciation; consonants omitted or substituted; which ones; slurring; dysarthria; nasality
   Are speech defects consistent or variable?

8. *Phonation* and volume of speech

9. *Prosody*: pattern of stress and tonal variation in speech

10. *Rhythm*: abnormalities of rhythm – stuttering, lack of cadence and inflection; coordination with breathing

Schools Which schools has the child attended? How did they get on? Why were they changed? Has any teacher ever expressed concern to the parents? Has any statement of special education needs been made? Does the child like the current school? Are progress reports satisfactory? Has the parent seen the child's teacher? (*See below on information from schools.*)

Sex Is there interest in the opposite sex? Has there yet been the development of menarche, body hair, or masturbation? Have they been instructed about sex, asked questions or had any sexual experience? Is there any inappropriate sexual behaviour?

Strengths What are the child's good qualities, abilities, and attractive attributes?

Temperamental or personality attributes

It is not easy to disentangle the child's premorbid characteristics from the present problems, but an attempt should be made. Some aspects of temperament are best shown in the response to new situations, new events, and new people, but attention should also be paid to mode of functioning in routine situations.

Meeting new people What is the child's behaviour with adults? With children? Do they go up to strangers? Are they shy or clinging? How quickly do they adapt to someone new?

New situations How do they react to new places, new gadgets, and new foods? Do they explore or hang back? How quick are they to adapt?

Emotional expression How vigorous is the child in expressing their feelings? Do they whimper or howl? Chuckle or roar with laughter? How happy or miserable were they before the present problems? How do they show their feelings?

Affection and relationships Is the child affectionate? Do they confide in anybody, and, if so, who? What friendships have they formed?

Sensitivity How do they respond to a person or animal being hurt? What is their reaction if they have done something wrong?

Information from school and other sources outside the family

Parental consent should always be obtained to contact any agency other than the referrer and the family doctor. In medicolegal work, consent is needed to contact any agency other than the referrer. Permission to contact the school and other involved agencies can be requested when the first appointment is sent. If permission is not given for a key contact, such as that with the family doctor, then it needs to be sought with detailed discussion and explanation of its importance.

A teacher's account of the child's behaviour at school is indispensable. Ask for information about:

- Attendance.
- Academic strengths and weaknesses.
- Non-academic skills (e.g. art, music, woodwork, sports, etc.).
- Behaviour in the classroom and playground.

- Social relationships with teachers and peers.
- Any other observations of importance.

For preschool children, a report along the same lines from a nursery or playgroup leader is of similar importance. It can be helpful to have this information available at the first assessment.

It is good practice to explain to the family that a letter will be sent to the family doctor after the assessment and request made to obtain old medical records, etc. The family doctor frequently possesses further essential information. In medicolegal work the final report will be sent only to the referrer, who will then distribute it to the appropriate parties.

Psychological testing is usually an important part of the systematic assessment of a child and usually provides quantified information from behaviour and performance in a rigorously controlled setting. Such an assessment needs to be interpreted in the light of the validity of the test and the nature of the problem. A low test score from an uncooperative child should not necessarily be taken as implying a limitation of intellectual potential. A normal or high IQ score in a child with problems in everyday learning does not necessarily entail a non-cognitive explanation: there may be impairment in aspects of cognition that are not assessed by the tests used. If the clinical appraisal of cognitive functioning is discrepant with the psychometric evaluation, then further enquiry is needed to find out why.

Synthesizing different sources

Evidence often conflicts. There is no single rule for how to resolve disagreements; clinical judgement is required.

When there is disagreement, first evaluate whether any of the sources is likely to be unreliable. Is the mother depressed and exaggerating psychopathology, or fearful of the consequences of the assessment and suppressing problems? Have the parents read accounts of disorders such as autism and presented a 'textbook' account? Does a teacher have insufficient acquaintance with the child to be accurate?

Next, consider whether disagreement comes from varying standards about what is expected from a child. Care-givers vary greatly in their beliefs about the degree of deviance that is required before they decide that a problem is present. It will not be enough to establish that a parent considers, for example, that their child is hyperactive. Rather, detailed enquiry will be needed to establish actual behaviours such as the length of time for which the child engages in constructive activities, and the time for which they can remain still in a situation where this is expected. Parents are often much better at the recall of details of behaviour than at the judgement of what is the range of normality, so apparent disagreements may disappear on close enquiry.

For some problems, priority should be given to one source of information. Children describe their depressed feelings more frequently than adults recognize them. Parental account may therefore be insensitive, and the rule is often adopted that the symptom of depression is present if *any* informant gives a clear account of a marked problem in the child. By contrast, antisocial conduct may be denied by the child, especially if parents are present, so that the parental account is often more sensitive.

For many problems, accounts may differ because the child is different in different situations. This specificity to context is in itself important diagnostic information; for example, hyperactivity that is pervasive across all sources of information is more likely to be based on neurodevelopmental dysfunction than the same behaviour that is seen in only one setting, such as school.

Finally, if doubt persists after careful enquiry and consideration of possible reasons, the best way of resolving disagreements is for the psychiatrist to make observations directly in the natural settings.

The assessment of children with developmental disorders

It is usually most convenient to begin with a chronological account of development. Rather than go immediately to questions of pregnancy and delivery, however, it may be preferable to start by asking the parents when they first became concerned that something might be not quite right with the child's development, and what it was that aroused their concern at the time. Particularly with a first child, the parents' concern may have been aroused long after the child first showed delays or distortions in development. It is helpful to enquire whether, with hindsight, the parents think that all was well before they first became concerned and, if not, what it was that might have been abnormal. Having established the time and nature of those first indications of concern, it is generally easiest to go back to the time of pregnancy and to work forward systematically up to the present time. Most parents do not remember at all accurately when milestones occurred if they were within the normal range, but they are more likely to recall them if they were delayed. It is helpful to focus on that aspect first before going on to tie down the time more exactly. When seeking to date milestones, reference should be made to familiar landmarks rather than to actual ages. It might be appropriate, for example, to ask whether the child was walking on their first birthday, or when they moved house, or at the time of their first Christmas, or when the second child was born.

Particular attention needs to be paid to the developmental aspects of play, socialization, and language. With respect to the milestones of language it is crucial to be quite specific about what is being asked. Parents are very inclined to interpret all manner of sounds as speech, and especially as 'mama' and 'dada'. Consequently, it may be wise to ask very focused questions such as 'When did she first use simple words with meaning—that is words other than mama and dada?',

'What were his first words?', and 'How did she show that she knew their meaning?'. In addition to the first use of single words, it is important to ask about babble, the use of two- or three-word phrases, the use of pointing, gesture, or mime, the following of instructions, and immediate or delayed echoing. It is helpful to identify some occasions that the parents remember reasonably clearly and then to focus on what the child was like at that time. In doing so, an attempt should be made to determine what the child was like at about 2 years, 30 months, 3 years, and 4 years.

Few parents think of socialization in terms of milestones or indeed in terms of specific behaviours. As a result, although the topic may be introduced by some general question such as 'How affectionate was he as a toddler?', it will always be necessary to proceed with a series of focused questions directed at eliciting information in key aspects of social relationships and social responsiveness at particular ages. Thus, for the 6–12-month age period it would be necessary to ask whether the child turned to look the parents directly in the face when they spoke to him, whether the child put up arms to be lifted, whether they nestled close when held, whether they protested when left, whether they laughed and chortled in response to parental overtures, whether they were comforted by being picked up and cuddled, and whether they were wary of strangers. Similarly with toddlers, questions should be asked about whether the child greeted a parent coming home; whether they sought to be cuddled when upset or hurt ('Did she come to you or did you have to go to her?'); whether they differentiated between parents and others to whom they went for comfort; whether they showed separation anxiety; and whether they could be playful and enter into the spirit of to and fro in a teasing or make-believing game.

Precise questions are required to elicit an adequate account of the child's play at particular ages. Thus, to determine whether play was normal at age 2 years, the clinician should ask about the child's use of toys and other objects. Did he or she recognize the appropriate use of miniature toys (e.g. by pushing toy cars along the floor making car noises) or rather did they tend to spin the wheels, feel the texture of the paint, or listen to the sound of a wind-up car? Was there any pretend play, as with the use of toy tea-sets, dolls, etc? Would the pretend play vary from day to day and would the pretend element be used to create any sort of sequence of story (with the toy cars racing each other, being parked in the garage, or being used to go to granny's home)?

Having obtained a history of the development of play, social interaction, and language—with special reference to the first 5 years—it is necessary to obtain a comparably specific account of the child's *current behaviour* in these areas of functioning. Before proceeding to direct questioning on particular features, it is helpful to get an overall picture of the child's activities by asking how he spends his time on return from school or at a weekend. Such a description usually provides a life-like portrayal of the bleakness or richness of the child's inner and outer world, and focuses attention on the activities and experiences to be asked about in greater detail. For adequate evaluation to be possible, the specific questioning should be based on a systematic scheme that ensures that each of the crucial areas is covered, as set out in Tables 3.2–3.3.

Table 3.2   Scheme for current social interaction

---

1. *Differentiation between people* as shown by different responses to mother, father, stranger, etc.
2. *Selective attachment*
   Source of security or comfort, to whom does child go when hurt?
   Greeting (e.g. parent returning from work)
   Separation anxiety
3. *Social overtures*
   Frequency and circumstances; appropriateness to the situation
   Quality: visual gaze, facial expression, and enthusiasm
4. *Social responses*
   Frequency and circumstances
   Quality: eye-to-eye gaze, facial expression, and emotions
   Reciprocity: to and fro dialogue
5. *Social play*
   Playfulness
   Spontaneous imitation
   Co-operation and reciprocity, sharing
   Emotional expression
   Pleasure in the other person
   Humour
   Social excitement

Table 3.3   Scheme for current play

1. *Social aspects* (see Table 3.3)
2. *Cognitive level*
   Curiosity
   Understanding how things work
   Complexity: puzzles, drawing, rule following, inventiveness
   Imagination: pretend play, creativity, spontaneity, telling stories
3. *Content, type, and quality*
   Initiation
   Variable or stereotyped
   Unusual preoccupations
   Unusual object attachments
   Rituals and routines
   Resistance to change
   Stereotyped movements
   Interest in unusual aspects of people or objects
4. *Attention*
   Orientation to a new situation and a new toy
   Distractibility to extraneous stimuli
   Length of time playing with each toy, and frequency of
   change of activity
   Persistence versus leaving play activities unfinished
   Acceptance of, and persistence with, toys or activities introduced
   by the examiner

The mental state examination

This chapter deals with the mental state examination of adults (see below) and also includes special points concerning the examinations of the elderly (p. 65) and those with learning disability (p. 67). Special aspects of the examination—neuropsychiatric assessment of both adults and children, examination of those with epilepsy, catatonia or those who are mute or in a stupor—are considered in Chapters 5 and 8.

The mental state of adults

The mental state examination elicits a snapshot of a patient's behavioural and psychological functioning. Its description should record information elicited by examination during the interview *as well as other relevant observations* (e.g. those made elsewhere in the clinic or hospital). There are three aspects to interviewing: obtaining information, observing the patient in a two-person interaction, and giving support.

An attempt should always be made to put the patient at ease, as only too frequently patients fail to mention crucial information through fear or anxiety. By doing this, benefits above and beyond the collection of clinical information can be gained. For example, a well conducted interview provides a depressed or anxious patient with an opportunity to explain their problems to a doctor who, by asking about each symptom suffered, may be perceived to 'understand'. The mental state examination therefore provides the interviewer with an opportunity to develop a therapeutic relationship further, and offer empathy and support.

When describing the mental state of a patient, it is rarely useful to employ the terms 'normal' or 'abnormal' because these terms convey little. Instead, a description of the signs and symptoms elicited should be recorded under headings listed below. This will enable others to form clinical judgements as to the significance of the information gathered, and will also be useful for future reference.

Appearance and general behaviour

Few doctors are gifted with the descriptive talent of Charles Dickens but a decent portrayal of a patient's appearance and behaviour is within the abilities of most. The aim should be to give as complete, accurate, and life-like a description as possible of how the patient appears and what can be observed in his or her behaviour.

Describe the patient's physical characteristics and general behaviour; is it appropriate, bizarre, incongruous, or agitated? How do they spend the day? Consider personal self-care (cleanliness in general, hair, cosmetics, dress), eating, sleep, posture, and facial expression (depressed, elated, or anxious). Are they relaxed or tense and restless; slow, hesitant, or repetitive? How do they behave towards other patients, doctors, and nursing staff? Is they warm and open; or guarded, hostile, and threatening? Do they show good eye contact? Are they distractible, or unresponsive? Do they appear frightened or frightening? Do they respond abnormally to external events? Can their attention be held and diverted?

Does the patient appear over-emotional (are they dancing and singing, or withdrawn, tearful, and sullen; wringing hands with anxiety or relaxed; preoccupied and perplexed, or do they show little emotional expression)? Do they appear to be responding to hallucinations? Does their behaviour suggest disorientation? Specify orientation if doubtful. Do movements and attitudes have an apparent purpose or meaning? Describe any motor abnormalities such as gestures, grimaces, tics, mannerisms, stereotypes, waxy flexibility, slowness, tremor, and rigidity). Is there much or little activity? Does it vary during the day, is it spontaneous, or how is it provoked? If the patient is inactive, do they resist passive movements, obey commands, or indicate awareness at all? A detailed account of the appearance and behaviour of a catatonic, mute, or stuporose patient is especially valuable (these presentations are considered in detail in Chapter 5).

Speech

The **form** of the patient's utterances rather than their content is considered here. Do they say much or little, speak loudly or quietly, talk spontaneously or only in answer, slowly or quickly, hesitantly or promptly, to the point or wide of it, coherently, anxiously, discursively, loosely with interruptions, with sudden silences, with frequent changes of topic? Do they comment appropriately on events and things at hand, or use strange words or syntax, rhymes, puns, clang associations? How does the form of talk vary with its subject; is the patient monotonous or lyrical? ***Verbatim samples** of talk should be recorded to demonstrate any abnormalities* such as flight of ideas, thought block, derailments of thought, incoherence or drivelling, reiterations, perseveration, neologisms, paraphasias, etc. Samples of what the patient actually said are more useful than your opinion as to whether, for example, they employed neologisms Attach or include in the notes any examples of the patient's writing that appear abnormal.

Mood

The patient's appearance, motility, posture, and general behaviour as described above may give some indication of their mood. In addition, their answers to questions such as 'How do you feel in yourself?', 'What is your mood?', 'How about your spirits?', or similar inquiry should be recorded. Whenever depressive mood is suspected, specific enquiry should be made about the following: tearfulness, sadness, diurnal variation of mood, initial and middle insomnia, early morning wakening. Consider any suicidal ideas or plans, attitudes to the future, hopelessness, self-esteem, worthlessness, and guilt. Note any loss of appetite, weight, energy, motivation or libido, or constipation. Many variations of mood may be present, not merely happiness or sadness, for example such states as anxiety, fear, suspicion, or perplexity. Observe the constancy of the mood during the interview, those influences that change it and the appropriateness of the patient's apparent emotional state to what they say. Note evidence of flatness or lability of affect, and specify any indications that the patient is concealing their true feelings.

Symptoms and behaviours associated with mania (elevated mood, little need for sleep or food, excessive energy, reckless behaviour, initiation of multiple tasks without completion, distractibility) and anxiety (tremor, dry mouth, butterflies, blurred vision, sweating) should also be evaluated and recorded here.

Thought content

The **content** of the patient's thoughts rather than their form is considered here. The patient's answers to questions such as 'What do you see as your main worries?' should be summarized. Are there any morbid thoughts, anxieties, or preoccupations regarding the past, present, and future? Do worries interfere with concentration or sleep? Are there any phobias or obsessional ruminations, compulsions, or rituals?

Abnormal thoughts should be described comprehensively and their precipitants, mode of onset, duration, intrusiveness, frequency, congruity with mood, fixity, and effect upon the patient's functioning noted. The description given should be full enough to allow future readers to make their own decision as to whether the patient suffered from, for example, a phobia, obsessional rumination/compulsion, overvalued idea, idea of reference, or delusion (including delusions of passivity and thought possession), all of which should be recorded within this section.

This section should always include an evaluation of any thoughts of **harm towards self or others**. Should such thoughts be admitted, a detailed account of the patient's intent should be recorded, including; the onset, frequency, planning, preparation, and desire to harm. The patient should also be asked whether they believe they are capable of realizing these thoughts, and whether there are any factors that prevent them from completing the act.

Abnormal beliefs and interpretations of events

Specify the content, mode of onset, and degree of fixity of any unusual or abnormal beliefs:

- in relation to the environment (e.g. ideas of reference, misinterpretations or delusions; beliefs that they are being persecuted, that they are being treated in a special way, or are the subject of an experiment)
- in relation to the body (e.g. ideas or delusions of bodily change)
- in relation to the self (e.g. delusions of passivity, of influence, thought reading, or intrusion).

Abnormal experiences referred to environment, body, or self

Abnormalities in perception should be recorded here:

- *Environment*: Hallucinations or illusions—auditory, visual, olfactory, gustatory, or tactile, as well as feelings of familiarity or unfamiliarity, derealization, or déjà-vu.
- *Body*: Feelings of deadness, pain, or other alterations of bodily sensation, somatic hallucinations.
- *Self*: Depersonalization, awareness of disturbance in mechanism of thinking, or blocking, or retardation, autochthonous ideas, etc.

The source, content, vividness, reality, duration, and other characteristics of these experiences should be recorded, and also the time of occurrence (e.g. at night, when alone, when falling asleep, or awakening). Ascertain exacerbating or ameliorating factors as well as the patient's insight into the cause, as well as the significance and emotional impact, of any perceptual abnormality.

The cognitive state

This should be assessed briefly in every patient and related to their premorbid intelligence (see pp. 69–78). In younger patients who are not suspected of cerebral organic disease, the tests mentioned in the following notes for orientation, attention, concentration, and memory should be administered. For older patients, see the section on assessment of the elderly patient (p. 65). When cognitive impairment or cerebral disease is suspected, further tests need to be given from the schema for further examination of patients with suspected organic cerebral disease (Ch. 5, p. 68).

Orientation

If there is any reason to doubt the patient's orientation, record their answers to questions about their own name and identity, the place where they are, the time of day, the date.

Attention and concentration

Is the patient's attention easily aroused and sustained? Do they concentrate? Are they easily distracted? To test concentration and attention, ask the patient to tell the days or the months in reverse order, or do simple arithmetical problems requiring 'carrying over' (e.g. 112–25) or subtraction of serial 7 s from 100 (give answers and time taken). Give digits to repeat forwards, and then others to repeat backwards (delivered evenly and at 1-second intervals), and record how many the patient can reproduce in each direction.

Memory

In all cases memory should be assessed by comparing the patient's account of their life with that given by others, and by examining the patient's account for intrinsic evidence of gaps or inconsistencies. Special attention should be paid to memory for recent events, such as those of admission to hospital and happenings in the ward since. Where there is selective impairment of memory for special incidents, periods, or recent or remote happenings, this should be recorded in detail, and the patient's attitude to their forgetfulness and the things forgotten especially investigated. Record any evidence of confabulation or false memories. If the patient confabulates, is this spontaneous or in response to suggestion only? Retrograde and anterograde amnesia must be specified in detail in relation to head injury or epileptic phenomena.

Intelligence

The patient's expected intelligence should be gauged from their history, general knowledge, and educational and occupational record. Where this is unknown, simple tests for general information and grasp should be given, and an assessment made of the patient's experience and interests. An indirect measure of intelligence may also be obtained from assessing the patient's scholastic achievements by testing reading, spelling, and arithmetical abilities. A more objective measure can be obtained by using the Mill Hill and Progressive Matrices Tests from which an Intelligence Quotient (IQ) can be derived. Disorder should be suspected if a discrepancy is found between the results of these tests and the level of intelligence anticipated by assessing the patient's literacy and numeracy, or if performance measures are markedly inferior to verbal measures.

Patient's appraisal of illness, difficulties, and prospects

What is the patient's attitude to his or her present state? It is regarded as an illness, as 'physical', 'mental', or 'nervous', or as needing treatment? What does the patient attribute it to? Are they aware of any mistakes they have made spontaneously or in response to tests? How does the patient regard them and other details of the condition? How do they regard previous experiences, mental illnesses, etc.? Can they appreciate possible connections between their illness and stressful life situations, spontaneously or when suggested? Are these attitudes constructive or unconstructive, realistic or unrealistic? Is the patient's judgement good when discussing financial or domestic problems, etc.? What do they propose to do when they have left the hospital or clinic? What is the patient's attitude to supervision and care?

The interviewer's reaction to the patient

If it is appropriate, a brief account may be given of the way in which the interviewer is affected by the patient's behaviour. Did the patient arouse sympathy, concern, sadness, anxiety, irritation, frustration, impatience, or anger?

The elderly

Most older people have no objections to cognitive assessment when it is introduced with tact. It is helpful to start off by asking whether the patient has experienced any problems with memory and concentration (and, if so, whether this has bothered them and what sort of things they find they forget). After this, the cognitive assessment may make more sense. A useful preamble is as follows: 'I am going to ask a few questions about memory and concentration. Some of these may seem very easy and others might be quite difficult, but we need to ask everyone the same questions'.

Some patients with dementia are unwilling to undergo formal testing and respond with irritation, unexplained refusal, or bland replies such as: 'I don't pay attention to that sort of thing'. Such replies may be an attempt to camouflage an impairment and should be handled with tact. A reliable collateral history is invaluable in these situations.

Where the patient agrees to formal testing, a short cognitive screening test such as the Mini-Mental State Examination (MMSE) or Abbreviated Mental Test Score (AMTS) may be used (see Appendix 2). The MMSE can give an approximate idea of the severity of impairment in dementia, while a high score may provide evidence against substantial cognitive impairment. It may also be helpful in future assessments to have an idea of previous function (and it is therefore important that previous assessments are obtained wherever possible so as to put any current score in context).

Interpreting the scores on the AMTS and MMSE

(See Appendix 2 for the tests.)

It is vital to take previous education, levels of literacy, and sensory deficits into account when interpreting scores from these screening tests. For example, someone with high educational attainment may have clinically evident dementia and still achieve a maximum score on the MMSE. Unfortunately, both screening tests have poor cross-cultural validity and results should be interpreted with appropriate caution.

Scores of 6 or below on the AMTS indicate possible dementia and the need for a more formal assessment (unless the test is being used in primary care to assess progress in a patient with known dementia).

The MMSE was developed at John's Hopkins University for use in neurological patients but has since been validated in a wide variety of settings. A score of 23 or less is indicative of 'dementia'. The MMSE is sensitive to the effects of age, educational background, and socio-economic status. For patients aged over 70 years who left school before the cut point should be reduced by 3 points.

Cognitive screening tests such as the MMSE provide relatively little information concerning specific cognitive deficits such as impairment of memory or frontal lobe function. If cognitive impairment is suspected, a formal assessment should be carried out as outlined in Chapter 5.

Mood state

Some elderly patients with profound depression deny depressed mood but show other prominent symptoms such as anxiety, somatic or dissociative symptoms, or cognitive impairment.

Psychotic and behavioural problems

These are best elicited from an informant.

Physical examination

Many elderly patients suffer from concurrent physical illness, and a thorough physical examination should always be carried out. Special attention should be given to any signs of physical trauma, possibly occurring as a result of abuse.

Environment

If the patient is being assessed at home, some inspection of the home circumstances should be made. This is an important part of evaluating the degree of risk posed to the patient (and possibly others). Remember that self-neglect is not diagnostic of any particular disorder and can occur in severe functional illness as well as dementia.

- Is the dwelling in a good state of repair and decoration?
- Is it secure?

- Is the gas, electricity, and water connected?
- Is there adequate heating and lighting?
- Is the gas ever left on unlit?
- Is there evidence of the careless use of lighted cigarettes?
- Is the patient able to call for help if necessary (e.g. via a centralized alarm system)?
- Is there enough food in the home to make, at least, small snacks and hot drinks?
- Is there evidence of urinary or faecal incontinence?
- Are any pets well cared for?

Mild or moderate learning disability

By definition, a learning disabled person will have a degree of developmental delay. Detailed examination of the mental state is critical; this is not easy but much information can be gained by observation.

Mood disorders and psychoses may present initially as behavioural changes, for example over-activity in hypomania, social withdrawal in depression. Autistically disabled people usually become more inaccessible when depressed: they present as 'more autistic'.

Abnormal mental phenomena may be expressed in a fleeting and fragmentary manner; sustained observation is often necessary to allow any abnormalities to emerge. Do not waste time looking for specific syndromes.

Severe learning difficulties

For people with mild or moderate learning disability, the normal mental state examination can be applied. However, severe disability is often accompanied by a major impairment of communication. It is therefore necessary to eliminate pain or a physical illness as the precipitant of a behavioural crisis. The first sign of a developing physical or mental illness may be an exacerbation of pre-existing symptoms or behaviour. For example, at the onset of a mood disorder in an autistic person there may initially be just an exaggeration of the autistic features. Pre-existing handicap (e.g. speech impediment) may mask the expression of typical mental symptoms. In this case, check for secondary symptoms, such as vegetative features (sleep, appetite, weight, etc.) when depression is suspected. The mental state may be difficult to define in detail, in which case the diagnosis must be based upon a balance of probabilities.

All clinical notes should be signed and dated.

Neuropsychiatric assessment

History

This gives a longitudinal view of your patient's condition and usually provides the diagnosis; examination should be considered confirmatory. A minority of cases may give misleading presentations, especially in the early stages or where there is an abundance of non-organic features (i.e. in psychotic, conversion, or factitious disorders). The time course of the disorder is most helpful in aiding diagnosis; focus on the mode of onset (and antecedent conditions) and the progression (the duration and fluctuations) (Table 5.1).

Table 5.1 Time course and diagnosis of neuropsychiatric disorder

Time course	Diagnosis
Rapid decline and complete recovery	Transient ischaemic attack, epilepsy, transient global amnesia
Slow steady decline	Alzheimer's disease, Huntington's disease, Parkinson's disease, normal pressure hydrocephalus
Rapid steady decline	Encephalitis, brain tumour, raised intracranial pressure, cerebral abscess
Stepwise deterioration	Vascular dementia, multiple sclerosis
Diurnal variation	Myasthenia gravis
Static condition	Autism, Asperger's syndrome, cerebral palsy

Presenting complaint

When was change first noticed? Who noticed it first? How did it affect daily function? Reason for presentation to medical services? Effect of any intervention at that stage. Any precipitating or relieving factors?

A collateral history from an informant is crucial in confirming the onset and course of the disorder, particularly when there is suspicion of cognitive impairment or clouding of consciousness. This means discussions with family; friends; work colleagues; as well as professional staff who have had contact with your patient.

Family history

Any fits; memory problems; dementia; or other neurological disorder?

Personal history

- obstetric complications?
- delayed walking/talking or other milestones?
- any learning difficulties?
- educational attainment?
- performance decline at work?
- any occupational hazards (e.g. lead or solvents)?
- amount, frequency, mode of administration (e.g. intravenous) of recreational drugs consumed, including alcohol. Pattern of consumption over time.

Previous medical history (Table 5.2)

Is there a history of childhood infections, fits, or head injury? If any loss of consciousness, for how long, and what memory blanks before and after. Has the patient ever seen a neurologist or physician?

Prescribed medication (Table 5.3)

Has the patient suffered any side-effects?

Mental state examination

This begins when the patient enters the room and provides a cross-sectional view of their condition. Do not hurry the patient and note the degree of cooperation. If cognitive impairment seems to be present, move to a full cognitive examination rather than struggle to obtain the history. If there is an apparent decreased level of consciousness, use the Glasgow Coma Scale (best verbal and motor responses, and pupillary reflex) to monitor this.

Cognitive examination

Keep in mind premorbid intelligence.

Table 5.2 Organic disorders and their neuropsychiatric sequelae

Disorder	Sequelae
Epilepsy	Post-ictal, ictal, interictal psychosis, Todd's paresis
Head injury	Personality change, psychosis, post concussional syndrome
Connective tissue disease	Dementia, depression, psychosis
Thyroid disease	Anxiety, depression, dementia
Diabetes	Hypoglycaemic episodes, cerebrovascular events, dementia
Cardiovascular disease	Hypoxic delirium, sleep apnoea
Surgery or anaesthetic	Cognitive impairment from hypoxic episodes

Table 5.3 Drugs that contribute to neuropsychiatric disorder

Drug	Effects
Neuroleptics (except clozapine), antiemetics	Movement disorders
Lithium	Tremor, confusion, ataxia
Neuroleptics	NMS* (hyperthermia, rigidity, autonomic lability, decreased consciousness)
SSRIs, MAOIs, TCAs, Lithium	Serotonin syndrome (restlessness, altered mental state, hyperreflexia, tremor, fits, rigors, myoclonus)
Amphetamines, appetite suppressants	Anxiety, insomnia, psychosis
Steroids	Confusion, depression, psychosis
Benzodiazepines	Dependence, confusional state, ataxia, withdrawal syndrome
Amphetamines, cocaine, LSD	Psychosis
Alcohol	Dependence, withdrawal syndrome, Wernicke–Korsakoff syndrome, ataxia, peripheral neuropathy, decreased consciousness, dementia, head injury, acute or chronic subdural
Antiepileptics	Confusion, ataxia, psychosis (especially vigabatrin)

*neuroleptic malignant syndrome

Orientation

Disorientation is a key indication of cerebral dysfunction, reflecting alterations in the level of consciousness. Time disorientation is regarded as the hallmark of acute organic reactions.

- **Time, place and person**—Does the patient know who they are, where they are, and what the date and time of day is?

Attention and concentration

These test alertness and the capacity to control information processing in the brain. Along with tests for orientation, they are a means of evaluating the patient's level of conscious awareness.

- **Reciting backwards**—e.g. give reverse days of the week or spell WORLD backwards.
- **Serial 7s**—counting down from 100 in subtractions of 7.
- **Digit span recall** (forwards and backwards)—remember to deliver each digit in a monotone 1 second apart (average 7 forward).

Language ability

Dysarthria a difficulty in the mechanical production of speech should be assessed before **dysphasia,** which is the cortical partial failure of language function. **Receptive dysphasia** can be detected by asking the patient to point to surrounding objects, or to respond to a short series of verbal commands. You can test for **expressive dysphasia** by asking the patient to name everyday objects (**nominal dysphasia**) or write a sentence of their own choice. Don't forget to check handedness as 95% of right-handers and the majority of left-handers have relative language dominance in the left hemisphere.

Repetition

- '**West Register Street**' and '**no ifs, ands, or buts**'—this tests for *dysarthria* and the intactness of the connections between the input and output of speech.

Comprehension

- **Response to simple instructions**
  - (a) point correctly on command (e.g. surrounding objects)
  - (b) carry out simple orders on request (e.g. pick up an object, show tongue).
- **Response to complex instructions**—tear paper into three pieces (Marie's 3 paper test).

Word finding

- **Name both common and uncommon objects** (e.g. parts of a wrist watch, and other objects in the room)—this tests for nominal dysphasia (the reduced capacity to retrieve words used in everyday speech), which may be the only language disturbance. Note circumlocutions used to cover this deficit.

Reading
- Observe for content errors (also dysarthria and dysprosody).

Writing
- Test **ability to write spontaneously** and examine written productions for substitutions, perseverations, spelling errors, and letter reversals. Note that asking a patient to write something of what they have just read (e.g. news item) also tests their comprehension.

Memory
Amnesia (acquired memory dysfunction) is an abnormality of registering, storing, recalling, or recognizing information and events. **Focal amnestic states** can occur with relative preservation of other cognitive functions, which contrasts with **diffuse amnesic states**. All are qualitatively different from **psychogenic amnesias**. Memory failure is a particularly sensitive indicator of cerebral dysfunction. The patient may have deficits in explicit memory, with difficulty in conscious recollection, yet retain implicit (procedural/skills) knowledge. For example, they may be able to find their way around familiar surroundings but be unable to recollect (describe) their route.

Immediate memory span (or 'ultra-short-term-memory')
- **Digit repetition** (tested previously).

Recent events
- **Recall of the temporal sequence of events** (e.g. the events of the interview).

New learning
- **Name and address**

  Ask for immediate reproduction (testing **registration**) and record the answer verbatim (repeat if necessary). If one or more mistakes are made, the entire name and address should be provided again. Test **retrieval** 3–5 minutes later after interposing other cognitive tests, and again record the answer verbatim.

- **Recall (paired association): free and cued**

  Give patient a list of six to ten paired items (e.g. colour–blue, flower–daffodil) or use a simpler test of three-word recall, each word being categorically different (e.g. car, river, monkey).

Giving verbal cues when spontaneous recall fails is a test of storage. A retrieval deficit is suggested if the patient's performance improves. Information processing is also being tested, as thinking of semantic links facilitates recall. These tests are especially valuable with anxious or disturbed patients.

- **Babcock sentence**

Ask the patient to repeat a sentence appropriate to their intellectual level, for example:

- **Dull** (50% of 11 year olds): 'Yesterday we went for a ride in our car along the road that crosses the bridge'.
- **Dull–average** (50% of 13 year olds): 'The aeroplane made a careful landing in the space that had been prepared for it'.
- **Average** (50% of 15 year olds): 'The redheaded woodpeckers made a terrible fuss as they tried to drive the young away from the nest'.
- **Superior intelligence**: 'One thing a nation needs to become rich and great is a large secure supply of wood'.

Test the number of repetitions necessary for the accurate reproduction. (Three repetitions of a sentence such as these should allow word-perfect reproduction.)

General information

- **Semantic (conceptual) memory**—for instance, names of key personalities, well known dates, places and events both distant and current.
- **Episodic (personal) memory**—matters unique to the individual (e.g. name of examiner, what the examiner has asked since the interview began).

Non-verbal memory should be assessed by asking the patient to reproduce a simple figure such as a cross, or a clock face showing a specific time, after a 5-minute interval. Initial copying of the figure tests **constructional praxis** (see below), as well as registration.

Apraxia

Apraxia is the inability to perform a volitional act even though the peripheral motor system and sensorium are intact. It is rarely seen without dysphasia, except in the case of constructional dyspraxia.

- **Ability to imitate postures and make-believe movements** (e.g. wave goodbye).
- **Ask the patient to perform a complex coordinated sequence of actions** (e.g. fold a letter and put it in an envelope).

Ideomotor apraxia is the inability to carry out simple coordinated movement sequences on command, despite being able to carry out these actions spontaneously. **Ideational apraxia** is the inability to carry out a planned complex coordinated sequence, despite demonstrating an ability to carry out each individual component. **Constructional apraxia** has been tested by the drawing above. **Dressing apraxia** is evident from the informant or by asking the patient to dress. **Gait apraxia** is assessed by the tandem gait test (see neurological examination).

Table 5.4 Features of parietal lobe dysfunction

Type	Disorder	Effects
Dominant	Dysphasia	Receptive dysphasia
	Gerstmann's syndrome[a]	Finger agnosia, dyscalculia, right/left disorientation, agraphia
Non-dominant	Topographical disorientation[b]	Getting lost, inability to learn new routes
	Agnosias	Visuospatial agnosia[b]: inability to recognize from visually presented information
		Prosopagnosia[b]: inability to recognize faces (associated with posterior lesion)
	Apraxia	Constructional apraxia[b]: difficulty in copying visually presented model (e.g. three-dimensional cube)
	Body image disorder	Anosognosia[b]: failure to recognize a disabled limb
		Neglect[b]: patient pays no attention to one side (e.g. shaving one side of face, drawing clock with only half represented)

[a]Seen more often in Multiple Choice Questions than clinically.

[b]Not very well lateralized, but deficits more common and severe with right hemisphere damage.

Table 5.5 Associated neurological deficit with parietal lesions

Location	Deficit
Optic radiation	Homonymous lower quadrantanopia[a]
Sensory cortex	Contralateral disturbance (e.g. astereognosis, reduced discrimination)
Perceptual rivalry	Visual and sensory inattention

[a]Posterior lesion.

Visuospatial function

Agnosias are rare and complex disorders disorders of perceptual recognition. The individual is unable to understand the significance of sensory stimuli even though the sensory pathways and sensorium are intact. All modalities may be affected but visuospatial problems are more common.

- **Distance estimation between objects**—tests proportions.
- **Copy a diagram**—tests constructional ability.
- **Freehand drawing**—e.g. drawing a clock face with numbers.
- **Ability to describe an object and explain what it is**.

Visuospatial agnosia (broadly synonymous with constructional apraxia) and **hemi-neglect** will be shown by omissions in the images copied. **Visual object agnosia** (visual recognition failure) is present when the patient fails to identify objects by sight and fails to name them; i.e. they are unable to get the meaning of the object purely by looking at it (but can through other senses).

Astereognosia is the failure to identify three-dimensional form and is tested by placing a familiar object in the patient's hand (e.g. a key). **Agraphognosia** or **agraphaesthesia** is detected by tracing numbers on the palms with a retracted ball-pen, which the patient then fails to recognize.

Table 5.6 Features of temporal lobe dysfunction

Type	Disorder	Effects
Dominant	Receptive dysphasia	Language comprehension affected[b]; includes alexia and agraphia in posterior lesions
	Amnesic syndromes	Especially for verbal material
Non-dominant	Visuospatial deficits[a]	For example, objects (visual agnosia) and face recognition (prosopagnosia)
	Amusia	Difficulty with melody, cadence, and emotional content of music
	Amnesic syndromes	Especially for non-verbal material

[a]Not well lateralized, but deficits more common and severe with right hemisphere damage.

[b]Superior dominant.

Table 5.7 Associated neurological deficits with temporal lobe lesions

Location	Deficit
Auditory cortex	Cortical deafness
Optic radiation	Homonymous upper quadrantanopia

Table 5.8 Features of frontal lobe dysfunction

Function	Effects
Social behaviour	Disinhibition, distractability, slowed psychomotor activity[a]
Motivation, planning and initiating	Lack of drive[a], poor goal-setting and learning
Organizing and problem-solving	Errors of judgement, failure to anticipate, perseveration[a]
Adapting and shifting attention	Catastrophic response[a], inability to adapt to the unexpected[a]
Personality change[b]	Over-familiarity, tactlessness, empty fatuous euphoria[a], sexual indiscretion

[a]Characteristics that help differentiate from mania.

[b]Two subtypes are described: 'pseudo-depressive'—akinesia (lateral frontal)—and 'pseudo-psychopathic'—disinhibition (medial orbital).

Frontal lobe function

Evidence of frontal lobe damage would have been suggested by a history of behavioural disturbance, personality change, and 'executive dysfunction' (e.g. disturbance to planning and monitoring goal-directed behaviours). The validity and reliability of the following tests are not beyond dispute:

- **Verbal fluency**—ability to generate categorical lists, e.g. words beginning with the letter 'F' (FAS test: 10 words per letter in 1 minute is the average).
- **Motor sequencing** (Luria's fist–edge–palm test)—should be assessed by first demonstrating the sequence to the patient and then asking them to continue the imitation for at least 30 seconds. Remember to vary the sequence between left and right hands to avoid a learning effect, and that anxiety is the most common cause of errors. Observe for motor perseveration.

Table 5.9 Associated neurological deficit with frontal lesions

Location	Deficit
Broca's area	Expressive dysphasia, if dominant hemisphere
Precentral gyrus motor complex	Contralateral hemiplegia
Supplementary motor area	Paralysis of head and eye movement (head and eyes turn towards diseased side), present only in the acute stage of a lesion, compensation occurring after a few days
Paracentral lobule	Bowel and bladder dysfunction
Optic nerve	Ipsilateral optic atrophy (when associated with contralateral papilloedema = Foster–Kennedy syndrome)
Olfactory nerve	Anosmia

Table 5.10 Other less common frontal lobe tests

Test	Response
Primitive reflexes	
Grasp	Grasping of the contralateral hand on stroking the palm from the radial to ulnar side
Pout	Pouting of the lips, elicited by either stroking down the filtrum or gently tapping on a spatula placed over the lips
Palmo-mental	A 'wince' on stroking the ipsilateral thenar eminence
Alternate tapping	Ability to understand a simple tapped code and adapt when told that the rules have changed (e.g. ABABAB to AABBAABB)
Perseveration	Motor or verbal; inability to avoid repeating the last given action or word
Reciprocal coordination	Ability to use both hands simultaneously smoothly and quickly without example

- **Abstract thinking and conceptualisation**
  - (a) proverbs (e.g. 'People in glass houses shouldn't throw stones')
  - (b) difference between concepts (e.g. child and dwarf).
- **Cognitive estimates test** (e.g. largest object in a household room).

Occipital lobe lesions
These can lead to simple or complex visual hallucinations, as well as difficulties with visual recognition.

Corpus callosum lesions
Callosal disconnection syndromes and severe and rapid intellectual deterioration (anterior).

Diencephalic and brainstem lesions
Korsakoff-type amnesia (especially deep midline); rapidly **progressive dementia** with intellectual deterioration secondary to hydrocephalus; **frontal-type syndrome** (with better insight); hypersomnia; emotional lability; stupor; akinetic mutism; pseudobulbar palsy; hypothalamic disorders.

Neurological examination

The examination does not have to be arduous for either the doctor or the patient. A recommended neuropsychiatric screen is given below, rather than a formal head-to-toe neurological examination. Note **handedness** by watching the patient write; test right/left discrimination. Observation of **gait** is a good way of testing voluntary movement. Ask the patient to walk placing one foot in front of another, as though on a tightrope (**tandem gait test**).

Sitting or other resting posture allows observation of involuntary movements.

Reflexes can be quickly tested with a tendon hammer once the patient is sitting or recumbent. Hyper-reflexic tendon jerks are most commonly due to anxiety. An up-going (positive) plantar or **Babinski reflex** indicates an upper motor neuron lesion. The primitive reflexes are described in Table 5.10 above.

Testing of **power** and **sensation** may be performed if the history indicates a deficit. Peripheral neuropathy is probably the most common positive finding and may be due to diabetes, alcohol or lead poisoning.

For test of **cranial nerves,** see Table 5.13.

Table 5.11 Assessing stance and gait

Deficit	Appearance	Confirmatory signs	Neuropsychiatric associations
Hemiplegic	Arm and hand flexed and internally rotated	Increased tone, brisk reflexes, upgoing plantar	Depression is common following CVA (especially in anterior lesions?). Hemiplegias acquired in childhood may lead to preserved language function at the expense of visuospatial skills, regardless of lesion site
Parkinsonian	Stooped posture, reduced arm swing, bradykinesia, shuffling gait which improves with afferent input (e.g. walking with a friend)	'Lead pipe' rigidity and 'pill rolling' tremor, which combine to give 'cogwheeling'. Paucity of speech and facial expression	Drug-induced (where tremor uncommon) seen more than Parkinson's disease (PD). Personality change (obsessionality and hypochondriasis) said to characterize PD. Dementia: 10–15%; depression common but unrelated to stage of disease. Psychosis usually iatrogenic
Cerebellar	Wide-based stance and gait, slurred speech	Dysmetria (past pointing), intention tremor, nystagmus	Possible current intoxication (alcohol, lithium, anticonvulsants) or chronic damage (e.g. MS—look for pale discs, pyramidal signs) or alcoholism
Akathisia	Motor restlessness, inability to sit or stand still	Subjective sense of inner distress and motor tension	Present in 20–30% of patients on neuroleptics; often overlooked

Table 5.12 Assessing abnormal movements

Deficit	Appearance	Confirmatory signs	Neuropsychiatric associations
Choreiform	Rapid, irregular, dance-like, or jerky involuntary movements	Consider more detailed cognitive testing	Accompanying medical condition (e.g. SLE, pregnancy, thyrotoxicosis). Drug induced: OCP, neuroleptics, phenytoin. Basal ganglia vascular disease; neuroacanthocytosis; Huntington's disease
Tic disorders	Repeated jerky movements, mimicking normal actions and under some voluntary control	Ask about suppressibility and obsessive–compulsive phenomena	Common in children but reduce with age. Usually affect periocular muscles, face, neck, and shoulders. Gilles de la Tourette syndrome begins with simple tics, progressing to jumps, genuflexions, and hops. Vocal tics and coprolalia also seen later
Dystonic	Sustained muscular contractions cause repetitive twisting movements, or abnormal postures and bizarre gaits. May occur focally (e.g. writer's cramp; spasmodic torticollis)	Re-check medication history: neuroleptics, antiemetics, SSRIs, and lithium have been implicated	Acute dystonia rapidly relieved by anticholinergics. Tardive dystonia is difficult to treat and can be very disabling. Rarer causes include Wilson's disease (look for associated basal ganglia and liver disease) and Huntington's disease

Table 5.13 Assessing cranial nerve abnormalities

	Name	Test	Importance
I	Olfactory	Omit: can be asked about	May be impaired in Alzheimer's disease or frontal lobe lesions
II	Optic	Ask regarding acuity. Test fields by confrontation, both eyes at the same time: 'Which finger is wiggling?' Assess pupillary reaction to light and examine discs for swelling or atrophy	Important to detect a field defect as this may aid localization (see above). Hemianopia implies a contralateral hemisphere lesion. If visual inattention is present (simultaneous finger wiggling), check parietal lobe function
III, IV, & VI	Oculomotor, trochlear, and abducens	Ask patient to follow your finger slowly, left to right, up and down. Look to either side on command. Ask regarding diplopia	Ophthalmoplegias are part of Wernicke's encephalopathy. IIIrd nerve (eye down and out) and VIth nerve (eye cannot abduct) palsies seen following head injury. Acute IIIrd lesion suggests raised intracranial pressure
V	Trigeminal	Test sensation left and right on mandible, maxilla, and forehead. Ask patient to clench their jaw	Trigeminal neuralgia can occur after herpes zoster infection, and the excruciating pain may lead to suicide. Palliate with carbamazepine or antidepressants
VII	Facial	Observe facial symmetry	Beware paucity of facial expression in depression and parkinsonism
VIII	Auditory	No need to test formally	Congenital rubella may result in deafness (plus cataract and low IQ)
IX & X	Glossopharyngeal and vagus	Listen to the voice and inspect the palate as the patient says 'Ah'	Lesion here (lower motor neuron) results in a bulbar palsy which may be due to tumour; MND: myasthenia gravis, etc. Pseudobulbar palsy (bilateral upper motor neuron lesion de-afferenting the bulbar nuclei) leads to dysarthria, a slow tongue, and a brisk jaw jerk. Often accompanied by emotional lability and a gait apraxia (marche à petit pas)
XI	Spinal accessory nerve	Ask patient to shrug their shoulders	
XII	Hypoglossal	Inspect tongue at rest; ask patient to stick out tongue	

Source: Kopelman MD (1994) Structured psychiatric interview: assessment of the cognitive state. *British Journal of Hospital Medicine* **52**: 277–281.

Neurological screening of children aged over 5 years

Children with known physical conditions or a history suggestive of a physical condition (e.g. epilepsy) should have a full neurological examination rather than this short screen.

1. Inspect ordinary gait.

2. Ask child to mimic:

    (a) heel-toe walking

    (b) tiptoe walking (possible above 3 years, usually no associated movements above 8 years)

    (c) hopping on each leg (hopping begins at 3–4 years)

    (d) kicking a ball of paper.

3. Inspection, particularly of hands and face, for dysmorphic features.

4. Touch fingers in turn with thumb. Test finger–thumb coordination bilaterally. (Most 6 and some 5 year olds can do it. Mirror movements usually absent after 10 years).

5. Check for dysdiadochokinesis on rapidly alternating hand movements (pronation/supination 15 seconds each side).

6. Touch my finger. Repeat three times for each hand (possible above 3 years, with eyes shut above 7 years). Note tremor, consistent deviation.

7. Stand up, arms out, fingers spread for 20 seconds. Age 4 years upwards: look for choreiform (small, jerky, irregular) movements of fingers. Over age 6 years: eyes closed, mouth open, tongue out. Look for asymmetry and drift.

8. Close inspection of eyes including ocular movements. Visual fields to confrontation.

9. Check face and jaw movements and power—whistle, smile, blow out your cheeks. Note tongue movements, wiggle tongue, lick upper lip.

10. Child removes shoes and socks (check shoes for uneven wear):

    (a) check muscle power and tone in arms and legs

    (b) check tendon and plantar reflexes

    (c) check feet for dysmorphic features

    (d) measure head circumference and plot on percentile chart

    (e) measure height and weight, and plot on percentile chart

    (f) estimate pubertal status (Tanner stages described on reverse of percentile charts)

    (g) observe how child puts socks and shoes back on.

11. Test hearing:
    (a) name large toy at 1-metre distance in a quiet voice (laryngeal component)
    (b) name ball, doll, car, spoon, fork, brick, ship out of the child's field of vision.

12. Check visual acuity (well-lit Snellen charts).

If abnormalities are detected the child should have a complete medical history and a full neurological examination.

The mute or inaccessible patient

Definitions

Mutism is the inability or unwillingness to speak, resulting in the absence or marked paucity of verbal output. It may be isolated, but often occurs clustered with other disturbances of behaviour, level of consciousness, affect, motor disturbance, or thought processes, and may be due to organic or non-organic disorder. **Stupor** is a term used by neurologists to describe a stage on the continuum with comatose, implying reduced consciousness, but in common psychiatric terminology stupor constitutes preserved awareness with severe psychomotor inhibition. Mutism is invariably present in stupor. In general, these terms should not be used in isolation, but should be combined with a detailed description of the clinical features.

History

The history needs to be obtained from informants—relatives, key workers, neighbours, etc. In particular, the following should be established. How long has the patient been mute? Was the development sudden or gradual? Was there a stressful precipitant, or did the patient seem overly sad or happy in the prodrome? Is the mutism partial or complete? Is it specific to one situation (e.g. school)? Does any of the patient's behaviour seem odd or bizarre? How does the patient function in day-to-day life—eating, drinking, sleeping, continence, social activities, etc.? Is there a past history of psychiatric disorder, conversion disorder, neurological or medical illness? What drugs have been prescribed or taken?

Examination

A general examination of physical state—temperature, pulse, blood pressure, and state of hydration (look at the tongue)—should be undertaken. The presence of mutism also demands a full neurological examination, beginning with an assessment of the level of consciousness. An impaired level of consciousness, or the presence of focal neurological signs, should lead to prompt referral to a physician or neurologist.

In particular investigate whether the patient can articulate (by making lip movements or whispering) and phonate (by humming or coughing)? Take note of the eye movements. Is the patient watchful, making purposive movements implying awareness of surroundings? (Beware 'roving eyes' in the unconscious patient; however, if the patient is lying down and the examiner moves the patient's head, the stuporous patient will fixate on a particular point.) Are the eyes deviated to one side or another? (Eyes deviate away from a focal lesion, but towards an epileptiform focus during a seizure.) Does the patient with closed eyes resist opening? Is re-closure of the eyes slow and uniform, as occurs in the unconscious patient (this can not be simulated), or is there resistance?

Is communication possible by other means, such as writing or signing? Are there any attempts to speak? To what extent is comprehension affected? (Pure motor (Broca's) dysphasia is normally accompanied by frustrated attempts at communication, and comprehension is relatively intact.) Speech delay is evident in a substantial minority of children with elective mutism.

Mental state

Note the state of mental arousal and motor activity; is there associated motor retardation? What is indicated by facial expression: does the patient appear elated, anxious, frightened, sad, or angry? Describe any grimaces, gestures, or mannerisms. Is there any evidence of attempts at communication, or does the patient seem unconcerned by their state. For example, is there 'belle indifference'? Does the patient appear to be preoccupied, perhaps by hallucinations, ruminations, or paranoia?

Differential diagnosis of mutism

Psychiatric disorders

- **Psychotic disorder**: mutism may occur as a response to a delusional system in schizophrenia or as part of the negative symptoms in association with reduced drive.

- **Affective disorder**: mutism in depression may result in psychomotor retardation or nihilism, whereas in mania it may occur as part of a manic stupor.

- **Elective mutism**: this is most often seen in children, where there is emotionally determined selectivity in speaking; it is associated with social anxiety, withdrawal or sensitivity.

- **Pervasive developmental disorders**: the use of language is delayed and often idiosyncratic, although mutism is rare. It is accompanied by impairments in social interaction and in a restricted range of interests.

- **Obsessional slowness**: this may be accompanied by severely restricted speech output.

- **Somatoform/dissociative disorder**: in psychogenic dysphonia, the ability to phonate may help in differentiating it from an organic condition. Post-traumatic stress disorder may also be accompanied by mutism.
- **Factitious disorder**: this is rare, but may occur in situations where divulgence of information may be detrimental (e.g. with a pending court case).

Neurological disorders

- **Lesions of cortex**: (e.g. frontal, speech areas), brainstem (e.g. akinetic mutism 'coma vigil'—'locked-in syndrome'), basal ganglia (e.g. Parkinson's disease, Wilson's disease).
- **Infective**: e.g. herpes encephalitis, HIV-related disease.
- **Drugs**: e.g. neuroleptics (which may cause dystonic reactions involving tongue and jaw muscles, as well as torticollis, laryngeal spasm, and occulogyric crises), lithium, sedatives, antiepileptics.
- **Seizure related**: e.g. during or after complex partial seizures, absence attacks, partial status.
- **Deafness**: may give rise to speech delay in children and impaired production of speech.

Investigations

These should include haematology, biochemistry including blood sugar, toxin/drug screen, syphilis serology, endocrine screen, chest radiography, EEG (which may indicate localized epileptiform activity, although its absence does not necessarily exclude seizures), and brain imaging with CT or MRI.

Initial treatment

Once serious neurological disorder has been excluded, a period of observation is often valuable, although the presence of severe psychomotor retardation in depressive disorder, or manic stupor, may require urgent treatment and ECT should be considered. Treatment of dystonic reactions should be initiated quickly as this is frightening and painful for patients. Intravenous or intramuscular procyclidine is spectacularly effective.

The catatonic patient

Definition

Catatonia is a term that was originally associated with a variety of psychiatric illnesses, and later specifically with schizophrenia. It is currently recognized as a non-specific syndrome that occurs in a variety of organic states as well as in psychotic, affective, and somatoform psychiatric disorders. Catatonia is characterized by abnormal motor behaviour, with periods of hyperactivity and hypoactivity.

Mutism and stupor are common, and it is often associated with features such as posturing, waxy flexibility, negativism, impulsiveness, stereotypies, mannerisms, command automatisms, echopraxia, and echolalia.

History

The ability of the catatonic patient to give a history may be preserved, and history taking should then proceed along normal lines. More commonly, however, communication is impaired, and assessment must be undertaken as for the mute patient, questioning relevant informants. If communication is possible, the patient should be asked about any meaning attached to the postures adopted, which may lead to the uncovering of a delusional system, the degree to which the patient is distressed by the motor symptoms (it is important to distinguish from the mental and physical agitation of neuroleptic-induced akathisia), and whether passive movement is painful (which is often the case in waxy flexibility). Ask about previous episodes of catatonia, as well as past psychiatric history.

Examination

As with mutism, the presence of catatonia demands full physical examination. Patients may shift rapidly into a period of catatonic overactivity, which could render people close by in physical danger; therefore vigilance should be retained during examination. The catatonic patient is at risk of dehydration, rhabdomyolysis, sepsis, venous thrombosis, and pressure sores, and examination should pay particular attention to these factors, as well as excluding the organic causes of catatonia. The following phenomena should be elicited where possible:

- **Automatic obedience**: a robot-like response to any instruction, however silly.
- **Negativism**: a similarly stereotyped response, but the opposite of what was requested.
- **Waxy flexibility**: the patient's limbs can be moved slowly into a new posture passively, but return gradually to the previously sustained posture.
- **'Psychological pillow'**: on lying down, the patient's head remains held a few inches above the bed.
- **Ambitendence**: the patient begins to make a movement but, before completing it, begins to make the opposite movement.
- **Echolalia**: the patient repeats the examiner's words or phrases.
- **Echopraxia**: the patient repeats any movements made by the examiner.
- **Mannerisms**: repetitive goal-directed behaviour.
- **Stereotypies**: repetitive non-goal-directed behaviours.

Differential diagnosis

Psychiatric disorders

- **Affective disorder**: Depression is probably the commonest psychiatric cause of catatonia and is considerably more common than mania. It often develops slowly; therefore, the history may be particularly informative.
- **Schizophrenic disorder**: 'Catatonic schizophrenia' is relatively rare now in Western practice, although catatonic motor disorders (i.e. a part of the catatonic syndrome) are commonly seen in all subgroups of schizophrenia. Catatonia is a relatively common presentation of puerperal psychosis.
- **Obsessional slowness**: Catatonic features may be due to severe obsessive–compulsive disorder. Access to the typical mental state (with ruminations and obsessions) may be available with observation or from informant's history.
- **Somatoform/dissociative**: This is rare and requires both the absence of physical or functional psychiatric aetiology, as well as positive evidence of psychogenic causation.

Neurological disorders

- **Lesions of cortex**: (frontal and temporal lobes), brainstem, basal ganglia, limbic system, or diencephalon (e.g. tumour, cerebral thrombosis or haemorrhage, head injury, infective—including encephalitis lethargica and syphilis).
- **Drugs**: e.g. neuroleptics (neuroleptic malignant syndrome—catatonia with rigidity, and temperature/autonomic instability), lithium, morphine derivatives.
- **Toxins**: e.g. carbon monoxide poisoning, alcohol damage, ecstasy, alcohol.
- **Seizure related**: e.g. simple partial or complex partial seizures.
- **Systemic**: e.g. renal, hepatic failure, endocrine disorder, connective tissue disorders (particularly cerebral SLE).
- **Other**: e.g. acute intermittent or coproporphyria, vitamin deficiency.

In addition, there is a proportion of patients who present with recurrent catatonia and in whom no psychiatric or neurological disorder can be found. This subgroup seems to be familial, and spontaneous recovery is the general rule.

Investigations

These should include haematology, biochemistry including blood sugar, toxin/drug screen, syphilis serology, endocrine screen, chest radiography, EEG (which may indicate localized epileptiform activity, although its absence does not necessarily exclude seizures), and brain imaging with CT or MRI. In the case of diagnostic difficulty, abreaction may reverse the catatonia of the functional psychoses for a short time, allowing the emergence of 'hidden' psychopathology; the response to a single administration of ECT may also be useful diagnostically.

Initial treatment

Supportive treatment, including fluid and electrolyte replacement, antibiotics, and anticoagulation should be initiated where indicated. Once treatable neurological causes have been excluded, consideration should be given to the early or even emergency use of ECT, as patients are at risk of a number of physical complications. Benzodiazepines, intravenously and then orally, have been shown to be of value acutely while neuroleptics begin to take effect. Neuroleptic malignant syndrome should be considered a medical emergency, and advice should be sought urgently. Initial treatment is discontinuation of the neuroleptic, supportive treatment of autonomic and temperature regulation failure, and treatment with dantrolene, benzodiazepines, and dopamine agonists.

6

The formulation, the summary, and progress notes

A **summary** is a descriptive account of collected data—objective and impartial. In contrast, a **formulation** is a clinical opinion, weighing up the pros and cons of conflicting evidence, and leads to a diagnostic choice. An opinion inevitably implies a subjective viewpoint, by virtue of assigning relative importance to each piece of evidence; in doing so, both theoretical bias and past personal experiences invariably come into play. No matter how accurate the final verdict, an analysis is inextricably bounded up with subjective judgements and decisions. When assessing the same patient, two experts may produce two similar summaries but two different formulations with divergent conclusions. This is the fundamental difference: a summary is descriptive, whereas a formulation is analytical. A summary therefore calls for the qualities of thoroughness, restraint, and objectivity, whereas a formulation demands the composite skill of methodical thinking, incisive analysis, and intelligent presentation.

   Formulating a case with clarity and precision is probably the most testing yet challenging and crucial part of a psychiatric assessment. The skill of writing a good formulation depends on the ability to differentiate what are the merely incidental and circumstantial biographical details from what are the salient and discriminatory features that form the cornerstone of a clinical diagnosis. Certain features are discriminatory because they support one diagnosis as the more likely candidate and discount another diagnosis as less likely.

The formulation

A diagnosis involves a **nomothetic** (literally 'law giving') process. This means that all cases included within the identified category have one or more properties in common. By contrast the formulation is an **idiographic** process (literally 'picture of the individual'). This means that it includes the unique characteristics of each patient's case that are needed for the process of management. So, while nomothetic processes are the only way we can advance knowledge about diseases, we use idiographic methods to understand and study the individual.

The format of the formulation

The formulation follows a logical sequence.

Demographic data
Begin with the name, age, occupation, and marital status.

Descriptive formulation
Describe the nature of onset (e.g. acute or insidious), the total duration of the present illness, and the course (e.g. cyclic or deteriorating). Then list the main phenomena (i.e. symptoms and signs) that characterize the disorder. As you become more experienced you should try to be selective by featuring the phenomena that are most important, either because of their greater diagnostic specificity or because of their predominance in severity or duration. Avoid long lists of minor or transient symptoms and negative findings, but include those that help to exclude other possible diagnoses. These basic data are derived chiefly from the history of the present illness, the mental state, and physical examinations, and are used to determine the syndrome diagnosis in the next section. Note that this is not usually the place to bring in other aspects of the history—that comes later. If we know the diagnosis of a previous episode of mental illness, this should also be taken into account, but remember that the present disorder may not be connected and the diagnosis may be different.

Differential diagnosis
List in order of probability all diagnoses that should be considered and include any disorders that you will wish to investigate. These will usually be syndrome diagnoses based on the descriptive formulation above. Give the evidence for and against each diagnosis that you consider. Include any current physical illness that may account for some or all of the phenomena. A common error is to include, for example, thyroid function studies in the investigations without including thyroid disease in the differential diagnosis. If you think a condition is worth investigating, you are obviously including it in your differential diagnosis; if it is not worth mentioning, do not bother to investigate it.

Remember that you will frequently need to consider supplementary diagnoses in addition to the primary diagnosis, for example alcohol dependence in the patient presenting with delirium, or a personality disorder in a patient with an anxiety state.

Aetiology
The various factors that have contributed should be evident mainly from the family and personal histories, the history of previous illness, and the premorbid personality. It may be helpful to order aetiological factors by making reference to the biopsychosocial model of illness. This suggests that you organize the aetiological factors relevant to an individual presentation according to biological, social, and psychological factors, subdividing each domain into predisposing, precipitating, and perpetuating factors. Try to answer two questions: why has this patient developed this particular disorder, and why has the disorder developed at this particular time?

Investigations
List all the investigations that are required to support your preferred diagnosis and to rule out the alternatives, and also list any that you think are required to improve your understanding of the aetiology. Give reasons for investigations if they are not self-evident. Remember that the thorough investigation of an illness requires effective enquiry into all the relevant domains of the biopsychosocial model; hence include psychological investigations as well as relevant social enquiry.

Treatment
Outline the treatment plan that you wish to follow. This should stem logically from your discussion of the aetiology as well as from the diagnosis.

Prognosis
Describe the expected outcome of management of this illness episode, with regard to both the symptoms and subsequent function (e.g. self-care and return to the community). Consider the risk of subsequent relapse.

The summary

This is an important document, which should be drawn up with care. Its purpose is to provide a concise description of all the important aspects of the case, to enable others who are unfamiliar with the patient to grasp the essential features of the problem without needing to search elsewhere for further information.

The first part should be completed within a week of admission and be arranged for typing under the following headings:

1. Reason for referral, and referrer

2. Present illness

3. Family history

4. Personal history
   (a) childhood
   (b) occupation(s)

    (c) marriage and children

    (d) premorbid personality

    (e) physical illness

    (f) previous mental illness

    (g) medication and treatment history

5. Physical examination

6. Mental state.

The summary of the psychiatric examination should cover all important aspects of the mental state and be drawn up under whichever of the subheadings in the main schema are necessary to achieve this. The six subheadings of personal history listed above should always be included, and others from the main schema introduced as appropriate.

The second part should be completed within 1 week of discharge and be laid out under the following headings:

- Investigations

- Treatment and progress—include details of medication prescribed and response; also note any significant side effects or reasons for changing medication. Document any other therapeutic strategies introduced. It is also helpful to document any significant episodes during the admission.

- Final diagnosis (or diagnoses) together with the diagnostic code number from the International Classification of Diseases (ICD), 10th edition.

- Prognosis—make a predictive statement related to symptoms and social adaptation, rather than terms such as guarded, good, or poor.

- Condition on discharge—include key worker, discharge medication and follow-up arrangements. Care plan (see pp. 178–9).

The completed summary should be short enough to occupy about 2 sides of A4 paper when typed. A summary is necessarily a compromise between the need to document all the significant aspects of an admission and economy. The summary of a readmission should include the full range of categories listed here, unless the last admission was very recent and it has been established that no significant change has occurred in the family history and personal history in the interim.

References to highly confidential matters (criminal acts, sexual revelations, etc.) should be included only if their omission would produce serious distortion of the overall picture. Often it will be preferable to include only a veiled reference followed by 'see notes' in brackets. The summary should identify which professional workers are to be responsible for different aspects of the patient's care in the future.

Progress notes

Regular progress notes, *signed and dated*, are a vital part of every case record. They should describe the treatment the patient is receiving (with dates of starting and finishing, and dosages of all drugs), significant changes in mental state, and any important events involving the patient. They should also record the opinions expressed by consultants at ward rounds and case conferences. In particular, you should record the reasons supporting significant changes in management. Although these notes must be sufficiently detailed to convey an accurate picture of the patient's treatment and their response to it, they should not normally contain lengthy verbatim accounts of conversations between patient and doctor. Notes that are excessively long are never read.

Handover notes

A *handover note* should be written whenever the patient is transferred from the care of one junior doctor to another, summarizing the salient features and outlining future plans. This is particularly important in the case of outpatients for whom there is no formal summary or formulation.

7

Special interview situations

The patient who demands proof that you care

Some very lonely people rely on their doctors and other professional attendants for social contact. Many of these accept the limitations and boundaries of the professional relationship and 'play the game' by generating the kinds of problems they know you deal with—side-effects of medication, new somatic complaints, etc. A small number make escalating demands based on the assertion that you don't really care—it is only a professional relationship to you. To demonstrate that you do care, you may find yourself putting them at the end of an outpatient clinic so that you can spend longer with them than with other patients. Then you may find that everyone else has gone home by the time you finish the consultation. As you recognize the person's really desperate state you may encourage them to phone you between appointments. Then, as it is clear that once-weekly visits to the clinic are insufficient, you find yourself offering extra appointments outside working hours. By this time you have a Very Special Patient, although often none of your tokens of care is having the desired effect. Far from the patient becoming happier and more able to face independent life, you are now apparently indispensable to their very survival. Indeed, suicide threats and gestures may be used to ensure that you remain centrally involved in the patient's care. Frightened, child-like behaviour may elicit an impulse to comfort the patient—holding hands, an arm round the shoulder. DON'T, you are in danger!

It is not that such people are not desperate and lonely and have not suffered terrible deprivation and cruelty in childhood. It is only that you will never be able to prove you care enough, not even if you were to adopt them into your own family. (Incredibly such things do happen.) The danger for you is that a central motivation in becoming a doctor—the relief of suffering and the wish to heal damaged minds and bodies—is being abused and your professional identity is under threat. Sexual contact between doctor and patient is far from uncommon and may happen as the result of a series of short steps, starting as outlined above. The contact can be heterosexual or homosexual, and it is an unequivocal breach of professional ethics.

The cardinal rule in caring for patients who demand proof that you care is not to feel that you should manage the situation on your own. The first step is to seek supervision from senior colleagues, and the second is to arrive at a care plan involving the multidisciplinary team. Ongoing supervision of such cases is essential to optimize care and to protect the carers.

The patient who solicits erotic involvement

From time to time a patient may develop an erotic attachment to the doctor and declare undying passion. Sometimes this can be managed by simply explaining that it is impossible for you to continue as the doctor if you are treated as a potential lover. Indeed, this may be the unconscious motivation of the patient's attraction, so that one could pose the question: 'What is it about my being your doctor that you wish to avoid?' Assessment of the underlying disturbance is essential, as such declarations may (among others) be the expression of extreme loneliness, the manifestation of a personality disorder, or the presentation of a potentially dangerous delusional disorder. Whereas you might try to work through the disturbance with the patient in the first two cases, this is not an option in the latter.

Whatever the disturbance, if the patient persists importunately, there is no alternative but to transfer care to a colleague, explaining that further contact between you and the patient will cease henceforth. Further harassment and stalking are matters for the forensic psychiatrist and possibly the police.

When such cases arise it is important to examine your own dress and behaviour to ensure that you are not unconsciously signalling availability or even behaving seductively towards the patient. A good rule of thumb is to seek supervision of such cases from a senior colleague and possibly a psychotherapist. It is important to record all interactions with the patient, by telephone or in the clinic, in the case notes. Each entry to be dated and signed.

The patient who brings gifts

In psychiatry one might expect expressions of gratitude less often than in other specialties. Nevertheless, patients do bring gifts from time to time. There is no problem with a parting gift at the end of a course of treatment: accept it graciously, unless it be cash. Gifts presented during the course of treatment are more complicated, and often contain a hidden message. Find a way of addressing this without being churlish; for instance, examples of work the patient has done (pottery in Occupational Therapy, a poem or a painting) may be important signs of competence and recovery; they may also be a concrete token of the patient's wish to remain in your mind and be part of your non-professional life. This is better put into words than left unspoken, and acceptance of the gift may be appropriate when the air has been cleared.

Ever more extravagant and inappropriate gifts might suggest that the patient has privately elevated you to a demi-god, to be placated, propitiated, and perhaps expecting one day untold benefits in return. This is a more direct attack on the professional relationship and needs to be addressed. 'I really cannot accept such an expensive gift. I wonder whether you fear I will not take you seriously if you come empty-handed?', or some variation on this.

The patient who is disinhibited

At its most harmless, disinhibition might take the form of personal remarks, tactless jokes, or asking personal questions. Do not rise to personal remarks or laugh at tactless jokes, and firmly fend off intrusive personal questions. In general, respond in a muted and subdued way rather than returning an inappropriate affective tone.

More difficult to deal with is the patient who enters your personal space, either to touch, stroke, or hit you. Depending on the patient's mental state, and with the milder forms of intrusion, you might try distraction, such as: 'You were telling me about the voices that you hear'. More overt intrusion is less easily dealt with, and you may have to withdraw and try again later, or return accompanied by a nurse. It is especially important to do this if the doctor is examining a sexually disinhibited patient of the other gender. Physical aggression calls for back-up, and you should always have access to an emergency button when seeing a potentially violent patient.

The patient who refuses to leave

Stand at the end of the consultation to signal firmly that it is over. Say, 'I am afraid I'm going to have to ask you to leave'.

Appeal to the person's better nature: 'If you don't go now, I will be keeping others waiting' (this, of course, may be the reason the patient will not leave). Finally, 'I am going to call for someone to escort you out of my room', and telephone for help. This is preferable to any attempt to coax or man-handle the patient on your own.

The patient out of hours

BE PREPARED and expect the unexpected: many awkward situations arise because the doctor has been only half-awake to the fact that psychiatric patients, at least from time to time, do not behave reasonably.

If you are called out of hours to see a patient you do not know on a ward or in the accident and emergency department, as far as possible inform yourself about them before the interview. Read the medical and nursing notes, especially the part I summary, formulations, care plans, and reports of management and ward round decisions. Ask to be briefed by the senior nurse on duty or by the accompanying friend or relative of the patient in casualty. Where possible, ask the nurse to be present while you interview the patient and never conduct a physical examination alone. If, for any reason, you decide to interview the patient on your own, first of all be clear how to call for help.

Position yourself within reach of the telephone—know the number to call for help. Be sure there is somebody within earshot who knows to respond quickly to raised voices or furniture being violently relocated. If there is a 'panic button', stay within reach of it. It is generally safer to position the patient nearer the door, leaving the path to the door uncluttered, as a paranoid or fearful patient is more likely to leave than attack if that possibility is open. If the patient produces a weapon, terminate the interview as quickly as possible by explaining that it is impossible for you to help them while they are armed, but that the consultation can be resumed once the patient has handed over the weapon to someone to look after it. Leave as soon as you have said this, if the patient will allow you to do so. Offer to get the patient a cup of tea or coffee while he or she thinks about what you have said. If the patient will not allow you to leave, stay calm, and chat about neutral matters; if you can press the panic button without risk to yourself, do so.

The patient who demands drugs

Often the story given is one of a lost prescription or of sudden motivation to stop illicit drug use. There are no rules about how to deal with this situation, but the following points may help:

- Take a good history of exactly which drugs and how much the patient is consuming.
- If they do claim to have lost a prescription, by whom was it prescribed? Can you check with them? Where is it being dispensed? Pharmacists keep good records and will often be open late.
- Do not prescribe unless you feel confident you are doing so safely.
- Never start a prescription that cannot be continued safely, for example by a local addiction service.

- Remember that opiate withdrawal is not physically dangerous, although benzodiazepine withdrawal and alcohol withdrawal can be.
- The patient has probably been using illicit drugs for a long time. They can continue for another day or two until an appropriate referral is made.
- Try to consult a specialist.

The patient who threatens violence

Even the most skilful clinician will occasionally be faced with a patient whose behaviour escalates such that physical assault seems imminent, or who even offers violence in so many words (but see Ch. 1, pp. 9–10). Usually, this arises when some real or perceived threat to the patient's physical or psychological integrity has made them very frightened and very angry—essentially, the patient feels that things are getting out of control. Particularly high-risk situations include interviewing patients whose delusional beliefs are that harm is imminent, or telling patients of a clinical decision to detain or treat them against their will. Patients who are disinhibited by drugs or alcohol are especially prone to sudden aggression.

Much can be done to defuse a crisis before violence erupts, and not just for your own benefit: other staff will avoid the risks of coming to your aid, and the patient will escape adverse labelling and possibly even a criminal conviction. Anticipate your interview with an unknown, possibly disturbed, patient by:

- reading the records for information about the patient's likely mental state and any previous history of violence and substance misuse.
- asking the nursing staff about the patient's current behaviour, concerns, and whether they think the patient has been drinking. Junior nursing staff will often defer to you on the question as to whether the patient is safe to interview alone (even if you know far less about the patient than they do)—unless you make it clear that you value their views.
- arranging to use an interview room that can be easily observed by staff who know where you are, or who are prepared to wait outside if necessary. The room should ideally have an alarm button that is close to hand, and the door should be easily opened from the inside. On the other hand, the room should also allow for a degree of privacy and quiet.

The interview itself should be conducted in a polite and, if anything, slightly formal manner. Not only will this promote a psychological distance between you that discourages violence, but, by treating the patient as someone important, you will increase their self-esteem. Do not invade their personal space, touch them, tower over them, or sit behind a large desk, but rather make an effort to build up rapport. Tell the patient who you are and that you want to do your best to help them. Take time to listen to the patient's concerns and, if they are delusional, acknowledge their fear, distress, or anger—rather than arguing about their veracity.

It often helps to tell the patient that they are frightening everyone, as they may genuinely be unaware of this. Similarly, asking a female relative or member of staff to sit in with you may help to modify the patient's behaviour.

With some patients these techniques will fail, especially if they have been drinking, have very fixed beliefs, or are very aroused. If your intuition tells you to be aware, listen to it. If you are clearly getting nowhere, do not increase the patient's frustration by prolonging the interview unnecessarily. Usually, the matter can be resolved only by telling the patient that you want them to do something, such as stay in hospital, take medication, or go into the seclusion room. By now, you will know that this is going to be provocative, and if you are alone with the patient it will usually be best to leave the room and fetch help; if necessary, tell the patient that you are going to consult a senior colleague. Confronting such a patient with medication should be done only with a control and restraint team in the room with you, and the medication prepared and ready to be administered.

The assessment of dangerousness

Recently, the general approach to the problem of 'dangerousness' has altered. The central focus has shifted from the question of whether a particular patient is or is not 'dangerous' to an assessment of the risk the patient poses in a particular situation under specific circumstances. This paradigm shift has facilitated clearer thinking about patients' potential dangerous behaviour in that it highlights the importance of psychiatric decision-taking, the information on which decisions are based, and their underlying logic.

Theoretical framework

1. Recognize that some level of risk is present
Just as the psychiatrist will automatically consider the likelihood of the patient committing suicide, so thinking about whether the patient may harm others must become routine. As with suicide, the risk of violence is sometimes unmistakable. On other occasions, however, it may be much less so. While apparently obvious, it needs to be stressed that recognition that the risk exists is the essential first step in the assessment of the likelihood of self-harm and violence to others.

In the case of suicide, actuarial data have helped to raise the question of risk in an individual by pointing to their membership of a vulnerable group. Similarly, the possibility of violent behaviour may be signalled by certain demographic and historical features of the patient's case—most importantly, a history of previous violence.

2. Define specific aspects of the risk(s)

Having become concerned that there is a risk, the psychiatrist should:

- define the risk and estimate the **seriousness** of the potential harm.

- make an estimate of the **probability** the risk will become reality.

- estimate the **imminence** that the risk will become reality.

3. Formulate a plan of management to reduce risk(s)

Such a plan will utilize the detailed account of the risk behaviour in terms of the nature of the act, circumstances, the victim(s), precipitating factors, and substance misuse to inform risk-reducing interventions. Note the importance of an explicit timescale.

Practical risk assessment

Assessments will vary according to the case and circumstances. Those undertaken to decide on transfer from a maximum-security hospital to a medium-security facility will differ from that carried out in the emergency clinic on an unknown man who has been behaving oddly in public. It is not only a question of the differing resources and information available. The purposes of the assessments, the relative urgency of the decisions to be taken, and the period for which such decisions will hold sway are completely distinct.

The practical process of risk assessment can be thought of as involving three stages: (1) gathering and reviewing all **documentation** from all possible sources; (2) **examining the patient** and **interviewing informants**; and (3) **asking yourself questions** about the patient, the circumstances, and potential victims. From the documentation and interviews, the psychiatrist aims to gain as complete as possible a picture of the index behaviour and its immediate antecedents, the patient's recent and longer-term history, the patient's social and physical environment (with recent changes), and the patient's mental state. Close attention should be paid to those areas where there are discrepancies between the patient's own account of their history and behaviour and the accounts of other observers, particularly involved family and nursing staff.

The index behaviour

Frequently, risk assessment is required for patients who have already been violent or have threatened violence. In such cases it is of the utmost importance to record a detailed account of the index behaviour and its antecedents. The patient will provide a partial picture, which may significantly minimize the violence. Any objective description is of great value, particularly witness statements recorded by the police. In addition to enabling analysis of the violent behaviour, witness statements often give a sharp and immediate sense of the emotional impact of the behaviour, an impact that is readily lost as the story is repeated through successive hospital admissions.

Such an account of the index behaviour may provide clues to the prevailing mental state, which are otherwise unavailable. Psychosis may be suggested by disorganized behaviour, apparent responding to halluci- nations, or bizarre actions. Patients may appear angry, afraid, or lacking in emotional response. Their actions may appear planned, impulsive, or a response to frustration or a shaming experience. They may have used a weapon defensively or with grossly excessive violence.

The immediate and medium-term antecedents

The immediate antecedents of the index violence may suggest precip- itating factors. The patient may have suffered or be threatened by the loss of someone important. They may have experienced rejection or loss of face. Their accommodation or financial security may be at risk. They may have refused medication or increased their misuse of drugs or alcohol. Evidence of relapse may be evident without obvious cause. A pattern of change may be evident in the patient's life culminating in the index offence. They may have become increasingly socially isolated and withdrawn, or have moved home ever more frequently, staying set- tled for increasingly short periods of time. Such 'social restlessness' has been seen as an ominous sign in the histories of particular psychotic perpetrators of irrational violence.

History from the patient

A comprehensive psychiatric history is an essential part of all risk assessments, with additional attention to certain specific domains.

Previous violent behaviour

Each incident of previous violent behaviour should be described. All behaviour bringing the patient into contact with the police should be ascertained, with the outcome recorded in terms of charge, convic- tion, and sentence including details of time spent in custody or on probation. Violent and criminal behaviour that did not come to police attention should also be recorded from as early as possible in the indi- vidual's life. So-called 'domestic' violence should not be neglected. Patterns, such as escalation in seriousness or decline in frequency, should be noted.

Exposure to violence

The patient's exposure to violence, both as victim and witness, should be documented from the earliest stage of their developmental history, as should include experiences 'in Care'. While the mechanism is ill understood, victims of abuse are at increased risk of becoming per- petrators in their turn as they utilize defence mechanisms such as identifying with the aggressor.

Psychiatric 'career'

The patient's psychiatric career should be reconstructed with attention to such factors as: mode of presentation; previous diagnostic formula- tions; whether admissions to hospital have been against the patient's will (under the Mental Health Act); the nature, efficacy, and time course of response to therapeutic intervention; and the various facets of insight including acceptance of medical explanations and advice, compliance with treatment, and spontaneously seeking psychiatric help. The success of outpatient management or the reasons for its failure are of particular importance. It may become clear that there is a constant relationship between psychiatric illness and violence and aggression or, on the other hand, that there is no relationship whatsoever.

Alcohol and drug misuse

The history of alcohol and drug misuse must be taken in detail, with particular attention to the relations between drug use and psychiatric illness, and between drug use and violence and aggression. These may be multiple and complex: violence when intoxicated may precede mental illness; drug use may exacerbate pre-existing psychotic symptoms associated with violence or precipitate relapse leading to violence; increased drug use may be an attempt by the patient to 'treat' their symptoms; criminal activity to finance a drug habit may follow loss of employment as a result of psychiatric illness.

Psychosexual and relationship history

The psychosexual and relationship history should be explored in detail. Childhood experience of sexual abuse significantly increases the chances that the adult will become a perpetrator. A pattern of short, unsuccessful intimate relationships may indicate one of a range of disorders of personality. Some understanding of attitudes to the opposite sex and sexual fantasies should be sought. Sexual psychopathology including dysfunction or abnormal sexual preference should be noted, especially if the latter has been acted upon outside a consensual relationship. Sexual partners are relatively frequent victims of severe violence associated with mental disorder, particularly if pathological jealousy is involved, and a pattern may be discernible over a series of relationships.

Circumstances

Thought should be given as to how the patient's situation contributed to the index behaviour. Who was he or she in contact with? Was the behaviour of friends or family a factor, for instance by encouraging drug or alcohol use or by discouraging compliance with treatment? Did the pattern of the patient's daily activities make the index behaviour more likely? Was the patient's accommodation appropriate?

The question of why the patient's victim was originally involved must be addressed. Was the victim a stranger, an acquaintance, or a family member? Was the victim selected as an individual, a member of a category, or at random?

Mental state

Just as a potentially suicidal patient should be asked about self-harm, so a potentially violent patient should be questioned explicitly about their intentions. The patient should be asked about specific victims (especially if threats have been made), methods, and plans.

Particularly associated with violence in psychosis are delusions of being under threat, of being controlled, and of having one's will over-ridden by some outside force. Acting on delusions is more likely if the delusions are associated with fear, suspicion, anger, or perplexity. Threats made by the patient must be taken seriously, as should violent fantasies. This applies as much to patients manifesting profound depression suggesting their families would be better off dead as to threats to kill uttered in anger.

The patient's insight should be examined in terms of their acceptance that they are ill, their agreement to take medication, and their understanding of the true nature of their psychotic experiences. Relative lack of conviction as to the truth of a delusion should not be seen as reassuring, because acting on false beliefs may be more likely if they are shakily rather than firmly held.

An exploration of the patient's inner world is as important as the clarification of external circumstances. The meaning of precipitating factors and the resultant violence to the patient is as important as the actual event. This is similar to finding out whether someone taking an overdose of what might seem a trivial amount actually thought it was a fatal dose. Complete denial of the index violence, or denial of personal responsibility for it, is of ominous significance, as is lack of remorse. The patient's attitude to any treatment received should be noted.

Relevant features of the patient's personality should be assessed. Personality strengths such as the ability to make friends or cope stoically with adversity may reduce risk. Deviousness or deceptiveness increases uncertainty. The damage to the personality seen frequently in schizophrenia may in some cases reduce the risk of violence by diminishing spontaneous activity. On the other hand, such patients' actions are more difficult to predict because of reduced access to their mental state.

Risk assessment: synthesis

Defining the seriousness of the potential harm, the probability that it will occur, and its imminence requires making sense of an often-considerable amount of information. Patterns should be sought in the patient's development as a child, adolescent, and adult that will contribute to a complex picture of the patient, their circumstances, and their interaction with potential victim(s). Prediction is facilitated by comparing and contrasting this picture with that of other patients with similar diagnoses, both known to the clinician personally and in the research literature.

Risk management

The purpose of risk assessment in psychiatry is the prevention of future harm by appropriate intervention. An effective strategy will change those aspects of the patient's situation and mental state which require changing and can be changed. It will also take account of important influences on behaviour, such as brain damage, which are not susceptible to intervention. Most importantly, the effects of each intervention should be monitored. Thus, long-term risk management involves a continuous process of assessment of risk followed by intervention followed by re-assessment of risk, which either confirms risk reduction or indicates that the intervention has been unsuccessful. In other words, patient management is continuously subject to *feedback monitoring*.

The multidisciplinary team should determine strategy and tactics for the management of patients who pose significant risk, especially by those individuals who will have specific roles in the patient's management. Success depends on the effective functioning of the team and on the *clear apportioning of responsibilities* within the team. Poor communication both within the team and between the team and other involved agencies has been held responsible for failures of management and the tragedies that have ensued.

Effective risk management involves breaking down a single large decision into a series of smaller steps. Thus, to decide that a given patient is unlikely to attack anyone before being seen in the clinic in a fortnight's time is a realistic possibility, whereas accurately predicting whether or not the patient will be safe in the indeterminate future is much less so. A patient's situation in the community in terms of friends and family as well as support services can be predicted reliably only in the short term.

Plans should be made to cover such eventualities as can be foreseen. These should be written down and known to the relevant members of the team. As stated above, all plans should include provision for effective monitoring so that both successful and failed interventions can be noted. Appropriate responses in the event of the failure should be spelt out clearly. It is obvious that risk management plans must take account of what is available locally, but it is equally obvious that plans may break down if a necessary minimum of community resources is not available.

Special problems

Childhood autism

Children and adults with autism or other autistic spectrum disorders demonstrate a combination of impairments in social relationships, communication, and the development of imaginative interests. The most distinctive aberrations are the difficulties they show in reciprocal social interaction, understanding the mental states of other people, sharing their interests, and forming friendships and intimate relationships. Their language lacks the usual social quality, and is preoccupied with idiosyncratic concerns. It may be lacking in quantity, for example used only to ask for needs to be met, or it may be plentiful but repetitive and more of a monologue than a conversation. Pronoun reversal (e.g. 'you' for 'me'), delayed echolalia, and stereotypical speech are common features when language is reasonably well developed.

(Immediate echolalia is seen, but is also very common in simple language delays and in children who are just learning to talk.) A restricted and repetitive range of interests and behaviours is very typical, and life may be dominated by incessant rituals, and by distress and rage if trivial aspects of daily routine or environment are changed. Partial forms of the disorder exist; the full form is usually very persistent. Long-term advice and supervision are needed, and families need support. Specialized educational resources can be recommended; behaviour therapy techniques can promote communicative development and reduce unacceptable and challenging behaviours.

Hyperkinetic disorder

This is a combination of impairments involving: an excess of activity, especially in situations expecting calm; inattentive and disorganized activity in every situation; and an 'impulsive' unwillingness to wait for gratification, share with others, or take one's turn. A multimodal treatment approach is usually needed in the management of this disorder, in order to promote academic and social learning, improve emotional adjustment and self-esteem, and relieve family distress. Behavioural approaches, with particular emphasis on speed of reinforcement, can be helpful both at home and in school. Drug treatment, especially with stimulants such as methylphenidate or dexamphetamine, is a powerful way of reducing hyperactive behaviour. Stimulant medication is therefore included in the treatment package of behavioural and educational support, in the case of children with severe hyperkinetic disorder.

Specific developmental disorders

These occur when there is an impairment of one or more developmental functions that is markedly out of keeping with the general level of development. For some functions there are reliable and valid tests that have norms for different ages: specific reading retardation, for example, occurs when performance on a standard reading test is worse than the fifth centile allowing for age and IQ, and it should be diagnosed by a psychologist's quantitative assessment. For other mental abilities (e.g. calculating) norms are much less satisfactory. For others again, such as motor delays and impairments of memory and attention, the diagnosis still has to be made on the basis of the clinical assessment. For all these problems, remedial education can be given once the problem has been recognized. Counselling for the child and family may be needed to help in the prevention of secondary psychiatric dysfunction. (See section on assessment of development, pp. 55–9.)

Suicide and deliberate self-harm

How common is suicide?

Suicidal behaviour is a major public health problem. According to the most recent World Health Organization (WHO) study on parasuicide conducted in 13 European countries including the UK, the average annual rates of suicide attempts are 136 per 100 000 for males and 186 per 100 000 for females. The rate of completed suicide in the UK is less than 10 per 100 000 per year, which accounts for 1% of all deaths. Suicide is the ninth leading cause of death among the general population in developed countries, and among adolescents it takes third place in the ranking of causes of death. Eight to ten people attempt suicide for every one who completes it, thus the lethality of self-harming behaviour is high. The adequate assessment, management, and ultimately prevention of suicide probably represent the most essential skill for a psychiatrist.

Useful definitions

The concept of 'suicidal behaviour' involves a continuum of behaviours ranging from suicidal thoughts to successful suicide. Full consensus on terminology has not yet been reached. The following definitions, based on ICD-10, are used in this book:

- **Suicide:** A willful self-inflicted life-threatening act, which has resulted in death.

- **Parasuicide:** A non-fatal act in which an individual deliberately causes self-injury or ingests a substance in excess of any prescribed or generally recognized therapeutic dose. The term **suicide attempt** is often used to refer to cases of parasuicide involving intention to die.

- **Deliberate self-harm (DSH):** A deliberate non-fatal act committed in the knowledge that it was potentially harmful and, in the case of drug overdose, that the amount taken was excessive.

The essential distinction is between those who commit suicide (completed suicide) and those who survive after harming themselves (parasuicide and deliberate self-harm). The challenge for the psychiatrist lies in the substantial overlap between the two.

Risk factors for suicide: features from the history that are associated with increased risk of suicide

The main risk factors are:

1. *A statement of intent:* About two-thirds of those who die by suicide have told someone about their intentions. It is a misconception that those who talk about suicide do not act upon it.

2. *History of previous suicide behaviour:* In the WHO multicentre study on parasuicide more than 40% of the sample had a history of at least one previous suicide attempt. Of all repeaters, nearly 20% made their second suicide attempt within 12 months of the first.

3. *Presence of psychiatric disorder:* Over 90% of victims of completed suicide were suffering from a psychiatric disorder at the time of committing suicide. The prevalence of psychiatric disorders among parasuicide cases is also very high. Disorders with a higher

risk of suicide are major depression, bipolar affective disorder, schizophrenia, and drug/alcohol dependence.

Further risk factors of suicide to remember and recognize include:

- Painful physical illness
- Bereavement
- Impulsive personality traits
- Social isolation
- Male sex
- Unemployment
- Low social class
- Older age (although risk is also increasing in young men)
- Previous history of DSH
- Certain professions (doctors, vets, farmers)
- Certain ethnic groups (Indian females).

Features associated with higher suicide risk (see also Table 8.1)

- Recurrent or persisting suicidal ideation (always remember to ask).
- Hopelessness
- Depression
- Agitation
- Early schizophrenia with retained insight (young patients who are aware of the implications of their illness and see their future ambitions restricted)
- Presence of delusions of control, poverty, and guilt.

Table 8.1 Features conveying a higher risk of repetition and eventual suicide

Higher risk	Lower risk
Previous parasuicide/DSH	First attempt
Attempt was planned	Impulsive attempt (not planned)
Attempt performed in isolation	Attempt performed in front of others
Precautions taken to avoid rescue	Rescue intervention likely or actively sought
Violent method (hanging, gun)	Non-violent method (overdose)
Patient expected fatal outcome	Patient unsure of outcome[a]
Regrets having been rescued	Relieved at being rescued
'Suicide note' or will written	No 'suicide note' or will written

[a]What matters is the patient's subjective intentions and expectations, irrespective of real medical seriousness.

- Being under the effects of alcohol or other substance (intoxication = decreased self-control = risk)
- Personality trait of impulsivity.

Systematic assessment of suicide/self-harm risk

The assessment is aimed at identifying subjects at risk, estimating the chances of suicidal ideas leading to acts, and estimating the chances of repetition of suicidal behaviours. Prevention is the goal.

1. The patient recovering from parasuicide/self-harm needs to be physically stable before you conduct a psychiatric assessment. Assessment of drowsy patients after an overdose is unreliable.

2. A first and crucial step is routinely making tactful but direct inquiries about patients' intentions. Asking about suicide does not make it more likely to happen. See page 3 for examples of key questions.

3. An essential part of the assessment is to determine the presence of any psychiatric disorder, i.e. to conduct a thorough mental state examination and take a psychiatric history.

4. All the risk factors discussed above need to be explored. There are scales to help you to do so systematically and a flexible use of those is recommended. See the 'SAD PERSONS scale' and the 'Risk-Rescue Rating Scale' in Appendix 3.

5. Identify any precipitating factors. Ask about life events, conflicts in areas of relationships, employment, finances, law/police, housing, sexual adjustment, physical health (especially HIV), and bereavement. Precipitating factors need to be addressed/resolved if further risk is to be prevented or decreased.

6. Finally, it is also necessary to evaluate the degree of support available in the environment of the patient. Assess the social support available and previous coping strategies. Could the patient's family or GP help?

7. If in doubt, always consult a more experienced colleague.

When these key aspects have been fully explored, a management plan will be established. When psychiatrists' interventions successfully prevent suicides no proof of efficacy exists, and often there is no acknowledgement; however, a completed suicide can be seen as a failure. This is not only an irony of our profession but also an increasing source of legal action. A practical advice is to write detailed records of your assessment in the notes and to monitor risk over time by making successive 'update assessments' for patients staying under your care. Systematic and careful assessments leading to sensible treatment plans and regular reviews of progress are the way forward. See page 108 and Appendix 3 for details on the management of suicide and self-harm.

Alcohol and drinking problems

Although acknowledged to be an important part of the psychiatric examination, the drinking history is often overlooked or patchy. Clinicians may feel that they are inadequately trained and too busy, or may perceive individuals with alcohol problems as 'too difficult' and time consuming. This view can be reinforced by the frequent attendance of severely alcohol-dependent individuals in crisis—intoxicated, aggressive, or suicidal. Taking an alcohol history is not the mere assimilation of facts. It is an opportunity to form a therapeutic relationship with the patient, to diffuse a difficult situation, and may even be helpful in itself.

Rather than confronting the patient with questions on quantity consumed and frequency of consumption at the outset—and risking a defensive reply—it may be more helpful to open with a non-specific question such as what they perceive as the main problem.

The alcohol history in the context of the background history

1. **Family history:** family attitudes to alcohol; whether alcohol was kept in the house; the drinking history of parents, significant others and siblings; family history of alcohol and other psychiatric problems.

2. **Personal history:** birth history and milestones; school attendance and performance; peer relationships; truancy; educational attainment.

3. **Occupational history:** what occupation—whether working with alcohol; occupational problems related to alcohol (dismissal, absenteeism, frequent job changes).

4. **Sexual and marital history:** sexual problems; history of childhood sexual abuse (particularly important in women with alcohol problems); HIV risk behaviour; marital problems related to drinking; separation; divorce; problems with children.

5. **Financial and housing history:** housing problems; rent arrears; eviction; problems with neighbours.

6. **Forensic history:** convictions for drink-driving, being drunk and disorderly, and violent behaviour.

7. **Past medical and psychiatric history:** particular attention should be paid to alcohol-related physical and psychological problems and accidents. Specific enquiry should be made for depressive illness, phobic anxiety, pathological jealousy, suicide attempts, and drug misuse.

8. **Basic personality:** ask the patient to describe what they were like before they developed their drinking problem.

Drinking history
Evolution of drinking and current alcohol consumption
Age of:
- first drink
- regular weekend drinking
- regular evening drinking
- regular lunchtime drinking
- early morning drinking.

Ascertain consumption at each stage, noting type of beverage and quantity consumed, as well as frequency. Note whether the person prefers to drink in a group, alone in a social setting, or alone at home. Note whether there is any binge drinking and detail any periods of abstinence.

Determine alcohol consumption (in units) for the past 24 hours, 6 months and 12 months (1 unit = 8–10 grams of alcohol = 1 glass of wine/half pint of ordinary strength beer/one measure of spirits)

Evolution of alcohol dependence   Note the age of onset of withdrawal symptoms and other features of the alcohol dependence syndrome (ICD-10):
- compulsion to drink
- difficulties in controlling alcohol consumption
- tolerance
- progressive neglect of alternative pleasures or interests
- persisting with drinking despite clear evidence of overtly harmful consequences

Alcohol-related problems
Outline physical, neuropsychiatric, and social problems.

Physical   Gastritis, hepatitis, cirrhosis, pancreatitis, peptic ulcer, oesophageal varices, oesophageal carcinoma, seizures, cognitive impairment, peripheral neuropathy, cerebellar degeneration, anaemia, cardiomyopathy, myopathy, head injury, etc.

Neuropsychiatric   Memory blackouts, pathological intoxication, delirium tremens, depression, phobic anxiety, suicide attempts, pathological jealousy, personality change, sexual dysfunction, auditory hallucinations during withdrawal, alcoholic hallucinosis, eating disorders.

Social   Marital, occupational, and financial problems. Forensic history.

A typical recent heavy drinking day
Most patients can identify a typical recent heavy drinking day. Some cannot, and this may imply more variability in their drinking with a tendency perhaps to weekend binge-drinking. Ask the patient to take

you through the day from the moment of wakening. A description of the timing and consumption of the first drink, and the patient's attitude towards it, can be extremely helpful in determining the degree of dependence. Thus, a man waking at 4.00 a.m., tremulous and drenched in sweat, who reaches out for the can of strong beer by the bed, is at a different stage of dependence from the person who takes their first drink at lunchtime. Likewise the professional woman who drinks covertly from a bottle of vodka in a workplace lavatory at 9.00 a.m. is at a different stage from the person who starts to drink at 5.00 p.m.

Other drug use
See next section.

Treatment history
GP; community alcohol team (statutory or voluntary); outpatient or inpatient treatment in general or psychiatric hospitals; residential rehabilitation; self-help group (Alcoholics Anonymous).

Drug dependence

When the answers to your screening questions, or other information (such as a routine urine drug screen), suggest that the patient has been using drugs, you will need to take a more detailed drug history. Below is a list of elements you will need to elicit, followed by a suggested schema and some suggested questions.

Important elements of the history

- Which drug(s) is the patient using?
- What is the frequency of use?
- What is the pattern of a typical drug-using day or week?
- What is the route of use (e.g. oral, smoked, snorted, injected)?
- What effect is the patient seeking when using the drug?
- Is there evidence of the physical or psychological features of dependence on the drug(s)?
- What risky behaviours does the patient engage in (e.g. injecting, sharing needles, unsafe sex, 'sex for drugs').
- How long is the history of drug use and how has it evolved?
- What complications of drug use has the patient experienced (physical, psychological, family, occupational, and legal problems)?
- What is the patient's past experience of treatment for a drug problem? Have there been any periods of abstinence and, if so, what has helped the patient to achieve this? What triggers have brought on relapses?

In addition, when you are taking a social history from the patient, assess the extent to which their main social contacts are other drug users or whether there are friends, family, or others who do not use drugs and who could provide support.

Suggested schema for drug history

Current drug use

Which drugs does the patient currently use? Ask the patient to describe his or her drug use the previous day, and to take you through a typical drug-using day (which drug, how often, which route). Ask also about the circumstances of the drug use: for example, some people will use drugs only in certain social circumstances (e.g. use of ecstasy at a dance party), while others may have a regular pattern of use that has developed to prevent the experience of withdrawal symptoms. Ask about a typical week if drugs are not used every day. Does the patient experience any withdrawal symptoms (ask the patient to describe them) or craving if the drug is not used? Ask about other symptoms of the dependence syndrome, such as increased tolerance to the drug, and the priority of drug seeking over other duties and pleasures. Is the patient currently engaging in any risky behaviour such as dangerous injecting (into groins or neck, or infected injection sites), sharing needles, or unsafe sex? How is he or she financing the drug use?

History of drug use

In addition to the current drug use, ask the patient whether he or she has used other drugs in the past. If the patient has used more than one drug, it is usually easier to take a chronological history of each drug in turn rather than try to assess all of them at once.

  Ask about the age at first use of the drug, then when the patient began to use the drug regularly. Ask about maximum frequency and amount used, and about any periods of abstinence. When (if ever) did the patient first experience withdrawal symptoms of the drug? (Ask the patient to describe them.) If not currently injecting, has the patient ever injected, and ever shared needles? Has the patient engaged in other risky behaviour (as above) in the past? What influences have helped the patient to achieve abstinence and then later to relapse?

Complications of drug use

Physical complications

Include complications of the drug itself and complications of the route of use. Ask specifically about hepatitis and HIV (e.g. 'Have you ever worried that you might have caught hepatitis or HIV?', 'Have you had any tests?'). Also ask about other complications of injecting such as abcesses, deep vein thrombosis, and septicaemia. Has the patient ever overdosed accidentally?

Psychological complications

Ask about the relationship of psychological symptoms to drug use. It may be difficult to tease out cause and effect, but some initial information will help in your assessment.

Family, occupational, and legal complications
Ask the patient about the effect of drug use on these areas of his or her life.

Treatment history

Ask about previous experiences of seeking help for a drug problem. Has the patient had help from a GP, drug dependency unit, or non-NHS organization? What has it involved; for example, has the patient had prescriptions, previous detoxification, psychological treatment, or self-help? What does the patient think was helpful in the past?

Current wishes and intentions
There are several possible goals in the treatment of drug misusers. Abstinence is one possible goal, but safer drug use may be a more realistic goal for some drug users (see section on harm reduction). Ask the patient what he or she would like to do about the drug use.

Special points in the physical examination

In the physical examination, look for injection sites, including legs and groins. If the patient is injecting, ask him or her to show you the most recent injection sites. Look for abcesses or infected sinuses, and for evidence of deep vein thrombosis.

Checklist of information

By the end of the history, you should have enough information to know:

• whether the patient is a dependent drug user
• what risks he or she is taking in relation to drug use
• whether there are current problems related to drug use.

Sexual and relationship problems

Sexual dysfunctions and desire disorders

History
This is taken from both partners separately, at least in part, but much of it can be usefully obtained from a joint interview, which also affords the possibility of direct observation of the couple.

• Features include the nature and duration of the problem—is it a disorder of desire or of function?
• When was the last successful experience?
• Does the problem occur in all situations (e.g. with other partners or in self-stimulation) or is it confined to the present relationship?
• Does it occur at all attempts; if not, what proportion of the time?
• Factors that seem to make it better or worse.

- Reaction of patient and partner when the problem occurs.
- Any associated difficulty (e.g. anorgasmia in the woman accompanying premature ejaculation).
- Attempts to treat the problem so far (both in therapy and by couple's own initiative).

Associated factors For example alcohol intake, smoking, spinal injuries, diabetes, hypertension, psychiatric illness and its medication, physical illness, surgical operations, stress, previous traumatic experiences (including sexual abuse or rape), recent life events, life-cycle stage, etc.

Quality of general relationship Communication, resentment, inhibitions, distance and closeness, invalidism, power, commitment. Any infidelities, satisfaction with sexual life, problems with fertility? Duration of present relationship, sexual preferences and practices, inhibitions? History from each partner, including sexual development, previous relationships and sexual experience, attitudes of family to sex, levels of knowledge, puberty, menarche, obstetric history, contraception, menopause, HRT, pelvic injuries or surgery, any sexual deviations, effects of ageing.

Full biographical and family history are often obtained via a self-report questionnaire before the couple is seen.

Masturbation Past and present—attitudes, guilt, fantasies, techniques, etc. Is orgasm achieved?

Physical examination
This is not always necessary, although it is usually recommended in cases of erectile disorder and vaginismus. Physical examinations should be conducted by a specialist, for example a urologist or the patient's gynaecologist.

Diagnostic features
Problems presenting in the male are:
- Erectile disorder (impotence)
- Premature ejaculation
- Delayed ejaculation
- Loss of desire.

Problems presenting in the female are:
- Vaginismus (painful spasmodic contraction of the muscles surrounding the vagina, usually impeding intercourse. It may be caused by fear or aversion to coitus but can also have organic aetiology)
- Orgasmic dysfunction
- Dyspareunia (pain during intercourse)
- Loss of desire.

Problems deriving from the relationship include:
- Incompatibility of sexual desire
- Conflict over sexual preferences and practices.

Direct questions should be asked about the presence of morning or night erections (suggesting a psychogenic aetiology), alcohol intake, use of drugs, sources of stress, any psychiatric problems, diabetes, hypertension, spinal injuries, pelvic injuries or operations, genito-urinary infections, etc.

There are no diagnostic tests that need to be done in cases of **ejaculatory or orgasmic dysfunction**, but medication with selective serotonin reuptake inhibitors (SSRIs) or other antidepressant drugs should be queried.

In **erectile dysfunction** there are some basic points that should be addressed. Enquiry should be made into the use of medication, including antidepressants, diuretics, gastric acid suppressants, and antihypertensives. Arterial blood pressure is a useful measure, as are reflexes in the lower limb and cremasteric reflexes, penile sensitivity, blood or urine sugar levels, and examination of the genitals. In erectile disorders the best source of information (if the test is available) is the intracavernosal injection of papaverine or prostaglandin: if an erection can be produced by this means it excludes vascular causes but leaves open the differentiation between psychogenic and neurogenic causation. This has to be determined on clinical grounds, but it is often necessary to assume a multifactorial causation. Further tests, including arteriography and cavernosography, should be reserved for cases where surgery is being contemplated.

For problems of sexual desire in men there is some benefit to be obtained from the measurement of hormone levels.

In cases of **vaginismus**, a digital examination of the vagina is necessary to make the diagnosis, but in many centres this is done at a visit later than the first, when the patient is more comfortable with the setting.

Sexual deviations and gender dysphoria

History
Denial is a common phenomenon in those with sexual deviations. In order to obtain a truthful account it is useful to ask open questions and to approach the topic in a roundabout way, for example when interviewing a man with tendencies to abuse children.

Details of the **deviant behaviour** should be taken:
- How often, where, when, with whom, whether caught and/or convicted, whether fantasies are associated, etc.
- What thoughts and feelings are experienced? What visual images or materials are used to achieve arousal? Does the person have a normal sexual outlet as well as the deviant one? What are the masturbatory fantasies?

- How high is the sexual drive (may be judged by masturbatory frequency or desired frequency of ejaculation)?
- How dangerous is the activity? Is it against the law? Does it damage the patient or others? Is there any empathy with possible victims?
- Do family members or partner know about the activities? What is their attitude?
- Past criminal history (this problem or others).
- Is the patient motivated by the wish to change their behaviour or simply to avoid punishment?
- Is there an associated sexual dysfunction in more 'normal' sexual activities?

Gender dysphoria   In cases of **gender dysphoria**, has there been a wish to be a member of the opposite sex from childhood, or is it more recent in origin? Has it occurred in the course of a depressive or psychotic illness? Has the patient thought through all the implications of sex change for themselves, their family and friends?

Diagnostic features
Variations and deviations can be divided into those that are harmful to others and those that are either solitary or harmless. Deviant sexual behaviour is predominantly a male problem, but it should be remembered that, especially with child abuse, women may also be perpetrators.

Harmful deviations include sexual abuse of children, whether general (paedophilia) or confined to family members (incest); rape (heterosexual or homosexual); indecent assault; exhibitionism; voyeurism; obscene telephone calls; stalking: frotteurism (touching people sexually in crowds); stealing clothing (to use fetishistically); and the more dangerous forms of sadomasochism including sex-murder.

Solitary deviations include cross-dressing for the purpose of sexual arousal; autoerotic asphyxia; and various forms of fetishism, including leather, rubber, shoes, underclothes, or different parts of the body such as feet. Relatively harmless deviations include cross-dressing for sexual arousal in the presence of the partner, the use of fetishistic objects with the partner, and some of the more benign forms of sadomasochism such as domination–submission, bondage, and spanking.

Trans-sexualism (trans-genderism)is not usually defined as a deviation, but is included here because there seems no more suitable place to discuss it. There are generally no biological abnormalities in these patients.

Couple relationship therapy

History
This is not usually a major part of couple therapy, and in some centres it is elicited by prior completion of a questionnaire by each partner.

What is required is a basic version of the general psychiatric history, including presenting problems and (for both partners) family history, personal history, previous relationships, current relationship, children, personality, and a brief symptom checklist.

In more psychodynamic settings the history comes out gradually in the course of therapy. Some systemic therapists spend time with 'genograms' or diagrammatic family trees in order to help in understanding family influences. In most clinics the therapist is as interested in the observed interaction of the couple in therapy as in the history as such.

In the couple interview, therapists will elicit details of the presenting problem, other strains in the relationship, the general satisfaction and commitment of both partners, the good aspects and troublesome aspects of the relationship, the risk of divorce or separation, problems with children, housing and financial problems, sexual satisfaction and what attracted them to each other.

Have there been major quarrels or violence? Infidelity? What are the resentments on both sides? Do they confide in each other? Who is more upset by the current problems?

Diagnostic features

These are more concerned with the couple relationship than with the individual, and involve such factors as closeness–distance, dominance–submission, alliances and boundaries, repetitive sequences of interaction, role-taking by each partner, relationships with other family members and outsiders.

Eating disorders

History

Many sufferers of eating disorders feel extremely ashamed about what they are doing and may find your questions very taxing and painful. Others are ambivalent about whether they want help; in some cases the denial is so extreme that they feel there is little or nothing wrong with them, and they have come to the clinic merely because of the extreme concern of their family or partner. Especially in the latter cases, it is important to establish an individual relationship with the patient rather than to relate exclusively to the family.

These patients arouse strong feelings, which range from anger and irritation through to the desire to rescue and protect. This is probably because their interpersonal schema includes a mixture of a drive to please others, a sense of inferiority, and a drive to be in control. One of the most important parts of the management is to understand this transference and countertransference.

Behavioural assessment

At the simplest behavioural level the clinician wants to know the following by the end of the assessment interview:

- Is severe undernutrition present or significant overweight?

- Is there constant dietary restriction and/or are there episodes of overeating?
- What weight control measures are used?

These behavioural criteria are easy to define and elicit, but they are also of clinical utility as they guide management.

Undernutrition or overweight?

This is addressed by measuring weight and height, and is usually done at the end of the interview with the physical examination (see below). A detailed lifetime weight and diet history is helpful. The patient should be asked when she first noticed a problem with her weight or when she first began to focus on weight as a topic of personal importance. Both the **rate** of weight loss and the **absolute level** are markers of dangerousness. Marked fluctuations suggest that there is self-induced vomiting or abuse of laxatives and diuretics.

The patient should be asked what her heaviest ever weight was, and when this occurred, and similarly about her lowest weight. The weight at which her periods began needs to be established, as does the weight at which her periods stopped (if relevant). This is important as the weight at which the patient's normal biological functions recover will generally be slightly above the former and so can give an indication of how much weight needs to be gained.

It is also useful to obtain a family weight history. There may be a strong family history of obesity in bulimia nervosa or of leanness or eating disorder in anorexia nervosa.

Constant dietary restriction and/or episodes of overeating?

It is often necessary to ask direct questions about bulimic behaviour as it may not be mentioned spontaneously because of the shame attached. A suitable line of enquiry is: 'Do you have episodes when your eating seems excessive or out of control?' You need to probe gently to elicit whether the amount eaten is excessive (objective binge greater than 1000 kilocalories) or not (subjective binge).

What weight control measures are used?

In addition to dietary restriction, the commonly employed methods are: self-induced vomiting, chewing and spitting, abuse of laxatives, diuretics, street drugs (e.g. amphetamines and ecstasy), caffeine, prescribed medication such as thyroxine, or health food preparations and excessive exercise.

Mental state assessment

Overvalued ideas about shape and weight, in which the assessment of self-worth is made exclusively in these terms, are considered primary features of bulimia nervosa. Not all patients with anorexia nervosa express such ideas.

Body image distortion (a statement that they are fat when they are underweight) is no longer regarded as a necessary criterion for anorexia nervosa. A less culturally bound description of this phenomenon is that the emaciated state is overvalued.

The patient should also be asked what weight she would ideally like to be. Often patients with anorexia nervosa try to please the therapist by giving a higher weight than they are aiming for. It may be helpful to probe into this in some detail: 'If you got to seven stone, would you be happy there?' If the patient says 'no', it can be helpful to press her as this may help her realize that she has a problem: 'So if you were seven stone you might want to weigh six and a half, but what then?'

Additional psychiatric disorders

More than 80% of subjects with eating disorders have additional psychiatric morbidity during the course of their life. Depression and obsessional symptoms are common in anorexia nervosa. Depression and anxiety disorders are common in bulimia. Symptoms of post-traumatic stress disorder are common in mixed anorexia nervosa and bulimia nervosa.

Personality disorders are present in half of patients referred to specialist centres.

Diagnostic features to look out for include:

- body mass index (BMI) of less than 17.5 kg/m^2
- use of weight control measures
- spot diagnosis—physical signs such as parotid or submandibular gland enlargement, eroded teeth, 'Russell's sign' callus on back of hand, cold blue hands, lanugo hair.

BMI can be calculated as follows:

$$\text{BMI} = \text{weight (in kilograms)}/\text{height}^2 \text{ (in metres)}.$$

For conversion of imperial and metric measures for weight and height, see Table 8.2.

Physical assessment

Nutrition

Many patients find it very difficult to allow themselves to be weighed. It is important not to get drawn into a battle over this, and the higher in weight the patient is the more lenient you can afford to be. The ICD-10 definition of anorexia nervosa requires that the BMI is less

Table 8.2 Conversion of imperial and metric measures for weight and height

	Imperial to metric	Metric to imperial
Weight	1 st = 6.35 kg	1 kg = 0.16 st
	1 lb = 0.45 kg	1 kg = 2.2 lb
	(1 st = 14 lb)	
Height	1 ft = 30.5 cm	1 m = 3.3 ft
	1 in = 2.54 cm	1 cm = 0.39 in
	(1 ft = 12 in)	(1 m = 100 cm)

that 17.5 kg/m^2 (this approximates well to the DSM-IV definition of 15% below average weight).

Cardiovascular system
The hands, feet, and nose are pinched, blue, and cold. In severe cases chilblains and, particularly in children, gangrene of the toes can occur. The pulse rate is slow (less than 60 per min) and blood pressure is low (90/60 mmHg). A marked fall in blood pressure on standing (postural drop) is evidence of dehydration.

Skin and hair
The skin is dry and downy, lanugo hair may be present on the cheeks, nape of the neck, and forearms and legs. The head hair may become thinned and dry so that it breaks off and sticks out. There may be a scar over the knuckles (Russell's sign), if the hand is used to induce vomiting. A petechial rash due to thrombocytopenia can occur with severe starvation.

Gastrointestinal system
Vomiting can lead to many physical consequences. The teeth may appear small and smooth with the upper front teeth worn into an arch shape; alternatively the teeth may be deceptively even if they have been crowned. The side of the mouth may be cracked. The face may appear rounded due to swelling of the salivary glands.

Skeletomuscular system
In severe cases a proximal myopathy develops. If this is present the patient may find lifting her arms to brush her hair difficult. She may not be able to get up without help or without leverage from her arms if you ask her to crouch. Tetany can develop because of the metabolic alkalosis (common in vomiting).

Somatization

Definition
Somatization is the term given when patients who fulfil criteria for a psychological disorder (usually depression and/or anxiety) instead believe they have a physical condition. This is a very common presentation of psychiatric disorder and is neither abnormal nor unusual. Somatization disorder refers to the most severe cases, and is a diagnostic category to describe patients who report large numbers of somatic symptoms, have illness histories stretching back to adolescence, and are very frequent users of medical services. The disorder is uncommon, but very demanding in terms of cost and time.

Taking a history from a patient with severe somatization can be difficult for psychiatrists. The intention is to obtain the usual information on the mental state, but without challenging the patient or becoming too 'psychological'. Thus, do not ask, 'Are you depressed?', but 'Has all this got you down?'. Do not ask, 'Do you feel like killing yourself?', but 'Have all your problems ever got too much for you?', and so on. Do not ask, 'Do you get panic attacks?', but instead probe about whether or not certain situations, such as supermarkets or the tube, make the patient worse. The patient who tells you they are made worse by neon lights, or whose 'brain gets overloaded by lots of conversations going on at once' may be experiencing phobic-related symptoms. Stress is a term that is often acceptable to patients when more direct psychological approaches fail.

One of the most important questions is, 'What do you think is wrong with you?'. The patient's illness model may explain much of their behaviour, as well as pointing to possible treatment avenues. Someone who is worried that when they get back pain their 'disc will slip again' and they will end up in a wheelchair will naturally restrict their activities. Many have similar 'catastrophic' cognitions: 'If I push myself I may never walk again, or I'll have a relapse'. Always ask, 'What might happen if you continued [when you get the pain … feel exhausted … feel dizzy]?' and 'What is the worst thing that might happen to you?'

History

The medical and family history of patients with chronic somatization can be revealing. A history of previous unexplained symptoms is common: tonsillitis persisting after the removal of tonsils, 'grumbling appendix', prolonged recovery from normal infections, repeated gynaecological procedures, and so on. Illness may also run in the family—looking after parents with long-term illnesses (either physical or psychological) is common. Previous episodes of ill-defined illnesses such as candida or unusual allergies are suggestive.

Always take a history of previous contacts with the medical profession; it is not advisable to criticize medical colleagues, but allow the patient to ventilate their distress at what may have been very unsatisfactory previous encounters.

Course

Somatization disorder is by definition a chronic condition. Patients attending specialist clinics with labels such as myalgic encephalopathy (ME) or chronic fatigue syndrome also have a gloomy outlook, associated with the strength of their physical illness convictions and the degree of avoidance behaviour.

Investigations

In general, most patients will have had more than enough investigations already. Once basic sensible investigations have been performed, further investigations will reinforce the sense that something organic is wrong. Investigations do not reassure such patients, and are anxiogenic, not anxiolytic. A better use of your time is to obtain as many medical records as you can.

Mother and baby problems

Pregnancy

Most general psychiatrists at some time or another will look after female patients who are pregnant, and a detailed assessment of the mother's mental health and adjustment may be necessary for a variety of purposes or reasons, as listed below. Maternal psychopathology in pregnancy is the same as psychopathology in other settings, and thus the principles of detailed history taking and systematic mental state evaluation are the same irrespective of childbearing status. The interviewer should, however, be sensitive to the fact that, in general, only a fortunate few expectant mothers conform to the stereotype of the pregnant woman who 'blooms' with good health, and for many women early pregnancy is a time of tiredness, appetite changes, nausea, loss of libido, etc. There may be anxieties and concerns about the future, doubts about readiness for parenthood, and uncertainties about the stability of key relationships, for example with the partner. Fears, ruminations, and fantasies about the fetus may have a bearing on the mother's mental state, but may not be mentioned unless asked about and then only if the mother has confidence in the interviewer.

What is the personal and social context of the pregnancy? Is it a first baby, have there been previous miscarriages and terminations? If it is a second or subsequent pregnancy, how old are the other children, are they in good health, and is the mother anticipating problems with the arrival of the new child? How much help and support does she have from family and friends, and how supportive is the expectant father financially, practically, and emotionally? What is his mental health like? Thus, the context of pregnancy imparts a particular focus to the psychiatric examination and, in terms of the mother's history, it becomes especially important to know what her own experience of being parented was like and what experience she has had of looking after babies and small children.

Clinically significant depression and anxiety is not uncommon in early pregnancy and may be missed unless specifically asked about. Clinical judgement is needed to distinguish between psychosomatic concomitants of depression and changes that occur in pregnancy. For example, can a woman who wakes up at night to micturate get back to sleep easily, does she wake feeling refreshed, is there a diurnal variation to her tiredness, and is her loss of appetite specific to certain kinds of food? How does *she* construe her physical symptoms, i.e. does she ascribe them to her pregnant condition?

Some important reasons for psychiatric examination in pregnancy

Termination of pregnancy

Abortion legislation varies greatly across nations and it is not possible to generalize about psychiatric indications. Suicidal risk and the possibility of severe postpartum destabilization of mental health are among the most prominent psychiatric considerations in countries with relatively restrictive abortion laws. There are no *absolute* psychiatric indications or contraindications to abortion; that is, apart from religious, moral, and legal considerations, there are no psychiatric illnesses or associated disorders (e.g. severe mental impairment) in which a woman's right to choose may be overruled on medical or psychiatric grounds.

Management of severe mental illness during pregnancy

Questions often arise about teratogenic effects of prescribed and non-prescribed drugs. What balance is there between the putative benefits of discontinuing medication and a flare-up of maternal illness? Clearly such questions can be addressed only in the light of a detailed knowledge of the woman's history and current state.

Welfare of the fetus and future safety of parenting of the newborn

Risks to the fetus may arise through infection, nutritional deficit, drug exposure, deliberate self-harm, and lack of compliance with antenatal care programmes. Thus, assessment of the mother's condition (e.g. chronic schizophrenia, eating disorder, drug dependence, personality disorder, depression, mental impairment, etc.) takes on an added urgency because of the risk to the unborn child, and this risk may enter the equation when assessing the need for compulsory treatment under the provisions of the Mental Health Act. Longer-term concerns about motivation and safety of parenting of the newborn should begin to be addressed during pregnancy in conjunction with social services. The psychiatrist may be asked to carry out an evaluation of the mother's mental illness, its history and prognosis, and her ability to manage her life in her personal and social context. There may be an inherent conflict between the mother's rights and wishes to be the primary carer of her baby and the paramount need to ensure the child's welfare and safety.

Prevention and management of postpartum recurrence

The likelihood of recurrence of severe mental illness (manic depressive and schizoaffective disorder, and possibly also paranoid psychosis) is high. Relapse rates of up to 50% are described and, therefore, it is negligent not to plan ahead by liaising with obstetric and primary healthcare services, and planning possible admission. Recurrence rates of non-psychotic depressive disorders are about 20%. Accurate and expert antenatal assessment by a psychiatrist is essential for planned management at a time when the mother is in repeated contact with clinical (obstetric and primary health care) services. Motivation to change may be a major factor in helping some expectant mothers to alter patterns of behaviour, for example of drug use and abuse.

After childbirth

The same general principles that applied to psychiatric examination in pregnancy also apply after birth of the child. Thus, some kinds of pre-existing mental illness have high rates of recurrence but, in addition, childbirth itself is a major factor in provoking first onsets of both psychotic and non-psychotic affective disorder. There are three conditions, the names of which suggest a specific association with childbirth: maternity blues, postnatal depression, and postpartum or puerperal psychosis.

Maternity blues

These are near universal, short-lived episodes of emotional lability, typically occurring around the fourth and fifth days after delivery. The commonest picture is of dysphoria, but this may in some instances be mingled with or dominated by elation, prolixity, and overactivity. The blues themselves do not constitute an illness or syndrome, and the two main points of clinical interest are the identification of the characteristics of those women who go on to develop postnatal depression and the distinction between the 'benign' self-limiting mood changes of the blues from the sinister prodromal symptoms of impending affective psychosis.

Postnatal depression

The symptoms of postnatal depression are the same as those of depression in other settings, but in addition the women frequently report ruminations of inadequacy and guilt about their ability to be good or competent mothers, and sometimes they describe feelings of aggression and impulses to harm the infant which are very rarely acted upon but which induce further self-blame. Thus the assessment of depression after childbirth should always incorporate sensitive questions about the mother's feelings concerning her baby and should extend to include obsessive ruminations and rituals as well as psychological and behavioural manifestations of anxiety, such as irrational fears, social and agoraphobic behaviours.

Postpartum or puerperal psychosis

These are affective (manic, mixed, or psychotic depressive) disorders, sometimes with paranoid, hallucinatory symptoms as well, which have an acute onset, usually at the end of the first or during the second week after delivery. They are commonly described as coming on after a 'lucid' period of a few days, and the affective illness is often very fluctuating and rapidly changing in its presentation with swings of mood and sometimes coexisting manic and depressive symptoms. In addition it is suggested that the presence of 'non-organic' confusion (i.e. perplexity and patchy disorientation) may be pathognomonic. It is entirely possible, however, that any subject who is in the early stages of acute psychotic breakdown may present in a similar way.

At the moment there are no treatments that are rationally based on aetiological hypotheses, and thus the choice of drugs is based on a judgement of the predominant clinical picture. Repeated assessments may be necessary, and too frequent changes of medication leading to poly-pharmacy should be avoided. Such assessments should also take into account possible risks to the infant if mother and baby are admitted together. Risks may arise through impulse in response to hallucinations or delusions, for example that the baby is evil and possessed, or that it is immortal and is an angel. Another major source of risk is through disorganization and neglect because the mother's interactions are too disturbed, for example if she is manic or agitated. Her interactions may be diminished because of intellectual impairment, or they may be inappropriate because she is chronically and severely impaired and lacking insight as part of a schizophrenic illness. In such circumstances the psychiatric examination must synthesize the doctor's own evaluation of the mother's mental state and behaviour, both alone and in the presence of the baby, with the observations of nurses and other members of the clinical team. Decisions about whether temporarily to nurse mother and baby separately may have to be backed by compulsion under the provisions of the Mental Health Act. Similarly, decisions about when it is safe to reunite them must depend upon the psychiatrist's assessment of the mother's mental state, her insight, and compliance with necessary restrictions.

Epilepsy and other neuropsychiatric syndromes

Epileptic seizures

These are classified by onset into generalized or partial seizures (clinical and EEG information facilitates this distinction).

Generalized epilepsy

- Absence ('petit mal') seizures, primary generalized ('tonic–clonic') seizures, and other seizures—myoclonic, tonic, clonic, atonic, and atypical.

Partial (focal) epilepsy with or without secondary generalization

- **Simple partial seizures** ('auras'): sensory, motor, or autonomic. Consciousness is retained. Auras vary in their complexity from discrete sensory experiences to complex ideation and emotion. Their pattern tends to be constant and has localizing value. They are abrupt in onset, intrusive, and experienced passively, and represent the portion of the seizure for which memory is retained.
- **Complex partial seizures** ('psychomotor seizures'): fugues, automatisms, and twilight state. Consciousness is disturbed at onset.

Epilepsy in childhood

History

Begin by asking for details of the **first attack** experienced by the child: age, circumstances, description, duration, how it was dealt with. Then ask for similar details about subsequent attacks.

Be careful to distinguish and obtain separate descriptions of all different kinds of attack. For each type of attack, probe regarding the following points.

Pre-ictal

1. **Precipitating events:** Are they through physical causes, illness, fever, etc.; psychological, any stress, or disturbance?

2. **Timing:** Do they occur at any particular time of day or night? How long since last meal, etc.?

3. **Altered behaviour or mental state before fit:** Is the patient irritable, restless, confused, apathetic, etc., minutes or hours before the attack?

4. **Patient's activity at onset:** Do they occur while asleep, on wakening, or in full consciousness? Are they precipitated by overbreathing, watching TV, walking out into bright sunlight, or any other change?

Ictal

1. **Aura:** What are the patient's subjective, warning experiences? Ask the child whether they know the seizure is coming and what they notice first (giddiness, noises, lights, smell, funny taste, inability to speak, feels frightened, etc). If the child cannot describe this experience, they may be able to draw it.

2. **Course:** What is the first event noticed (noises, strange behaviour, cry, fall to ground, motionless stare, etc.)?

3. **Posture during attack:** Did the child fall, go limp, remain standing, slump back in chair, etc.?

4. **Movements:** Which parts moved? One side or both? Synchronous or not? (e.g. turning of head or eyes, tonic stiffening movements, clonic jerking movements, restless or semi-purposive behaviour, automatic or repetitive acts, fumbling, mouth movements).

5. **Spread (march) of movements:** Where did the fit start? Did it spread anywhere?

6. **Consciousness:** Was the child totally unresponsive? Aware, but unable to talk? Fully conscious and talking?

7. **Colour changes:** Did the child become pale, flushed, or blue?

8. **Autonomic effects:** Examples include becoming hot and sweaty, cold and sweaty, or salivating.

9. **Incontinence:** Was there any incontinence of urine or faeces?

10. **Injury:** Was the tongue bitten or any other injury sustained?

Post-ictal

- **After-effects:** Did they return to normal immediately or go to sleep or become sleepy? Were they confused? Was there any weakness or paralysis of arms or legs? Clumsiness? Difficulty with speech? Change of behaviour or emotional state? Other symptoms, e.g. headache? Vomiting?

Duration and frequency of this type of fit   If not mentioned by parent, ask specifically regarding the following:

- **Generalized convulsive seizures**, e.g. are there ever attacks in which the child passes out completely? Are there movements of the arms or legs in any of these attacks—tonic–clonic or clonic–tonic–clonic?
- **Generalized absence seizures,** e.g. is there ever a momentary blank spell in which the child seems to be out of touch for a moment, but does not fall down, and for which there is no memory subsequently? Are there any movements at all whilst this is happening?
- **Other generalized attacks,** e.g. does the child ever make odd jerky movements (myoclonus)? Do they ever fall down suddenly without jerking or going stiff (drop attacks)?
- **Simple partial seizures,** e.g. are there any attacks in which there are movements of the arms or legs, but the child does not pass out or lose touch?
- **Complex partial seizures,** e.g. does the child ever have episodes in which they do not seem themselves or do peculiar things?
- **Reflex attacks,** e.g. does the child know how to stop an attack coming on? Ask the child privately whether he or she knows how to make an attack start.

Treatment

Is this by family doctor or paediatrician? Which drugs are used in what doses? (Calculate dose per kg per day—does it fall within the recommended range?) What side-effects are there? Have blood levels been measured recently? What do parents do during the attack?

Attitudes

Obtain parental attitude to the attacks. What did they think was happening during the first attack? What do they put them down to? What does the child put them down to?

Does the child have epilepsy?

1. **Differential diagnosis** includes syncope, breath-holding attacks, sleep disorder, benign paroxysmal vertigo.
2. **Pseudo-seizures** are more common in children who also have genuine seizures.

3. Remember **fictitious epilepsy** is not uncommon. Obtain the name of someone other than the parent who has witnessed an attack and who can be contacted (e.g. schoolteacher).

Notes

1. Children who are suspected or known to have seizures need a complete physical examination.

2. If the child is asked to count to 100, hesitations may reveal brief **absence seizures.**

3. **Starting anticonvulsants** is a serious decision. If there is still doubt about whether the child has seizures after a detailed history, consider asking the child to hyperventilate for 3 minutes. In susceptible children this procedure will induce generalized absence seizures in most, and complex partial seizures in a proportion. If a good history of generalized convulsive seizures has been obtained, there is no point in doing this test. In view of the potential danger, this procedure should be carried out only under careful supervision including the availability of drugs and equipment for the management of status epilepticus.

Epilepsy in adults

History

Ask the patient whether they have had a blackout recently, and when exactly?

Obtain a description of the attack. This should include a description by the patient complemented by a description from an informant who has witnessed an attack. The patient may have had more than one form of attack. Ask them to describe a typical attack from the beginning.

Pre-ictal   Can the patient (or close observer) predict that an attack will happen minutes or hours before it does? How?—change in mood (irritability, dysphoria); cognition (inattentiveness, confused behaviour); build-up of minor seizures (absences, myoclonic jerks). Do these features resolve once the attack has occurred?

The epileptic attack   The presence of aura indicates focal cortical onset and strongly suggests underlying brain damage or disease. Is there any immediate warning of the attack or does the patient lose consciousness abruptly. If there is a warning, for how long does it last? Does it last long enough to take avoiding action? Auras rarely exceed 1 minute in duration. Enquire after the aura content. Alimentary (epigastric sensations) and psychic (déjà vu, hallucinatory) auras suggest a temporal lobe focus. A sensorimotor 'march' suggests a primary sensorimotor cortical focus:

- Is consciousness lost suddenly or gradually?

- Is the patient completely unconscious or do they retain some awareness of what is going on around them? (If so, what?)

What were they told of how they were while unconscious? Do they fall or slump to the ground, or are they able to maintain their posture? Are they perfectly still or do they make movements? If the latter, are the movements rhythmic or irregular? Which parts of the body are involved? Are they more marked on one side of the body than the other? Is there any spread or are they generalized from the beginning? Is there any initial rotation of the head/eyes to one side?

· How long does this phase last?

If the patient retains posture:

· Do they carry out any automatism (coordinated movement—fumbling, searching, etc.)?

· Is there any tongue, lip, cheek biting or urinary incontinence?

After the patient appears to regain consciousness, how are they:

· Confused, sleepy, delayed speech recovery, quick recovery?

Are any other epileptic episodes described:

· Absences, myoclonic jerks?

Course   When was the first seizure? When was the patient first investigated? What was the patient and family told? When was the patient first started on anticonvulsants? What was the past seizure frequency, and present seizure frequency?

1. **Seizure pattern:** diurnal, nocturnal (how is this recognized), or both.

2. **Precipitating factors:** stress, menses, photic stimulation (self-induced flicker effect, TV, nightclub stroboscope), lack of sleep, non-compliance with medication.

3. **Predisposing factors:** family history of epilepsy, difficult birth, febrile fits during infancy, history of head injury, brain infection (meningitis, encephalitis), seizures following immunization.

Diagnostic features to look out for
Other diagnostic possibilities

· **Pseudo-seizures:** atypical features to the seizure—opisthotonos, pelvic thrusting, thrashing limbs, resists examination.

· **Panic disorder:** preceded by hyperventilation, chest discomfort, peripheral paraesthesiae, carpopedal spasm.

· **Alcohol related:** history of excessive alcohol consumption. Seizures occur during drinking bouts or immediately after withdrawal.

· **Other:** cardiac syncope, vasovagal episodes.

Differential diagnosis of confused behaviours occurring in the context of epilepsy

1. **Post-ictal psychosis:** follows exacerbation of seizure activity, post-ictal latent period of normality before psychotic symptoms begin, clinical picture dominated by confusion, hallucinations, and affective disturbance (twilight state), history of previous episodes; usually lasts only a few days and is self-limiting.

2. **Post-ictal confusion:** history of recent seizure, patient confused and drowsy; usually resolves within a couple of hours.

3. **Alcohol intoxication:** evident signs of drunken behaviour, alcohol on breath, known history.

4. **Head injury:** careful neurological examination indicated if recent history of head injury or evidence of scalp/facial injuries.

5. **Anticonvulsant medication:** complaints of drowsiness, poor coordination. On examination, nystagmus, dysarthria, and ataxia. There may be a history of recent change in drug dosage.

Immediate management
Related to epilepsy

1. If seizures are **well controlled**—find out from patient where epilepsy is treated and copy clinical correspondence with details of psychiatric diagnosis and treatment.

2. If seizures are **poorly controlled**—obtain details of medication, check compliance, request plasma anticonvulsant levels, and, once available, correspond as above.

3. Patient is **confused and disoriented**—this is usually due to post-ictal confusion, but see differential diagnosis of confused behaviours above. Post-ictal confusion will rarely exceed 6 hours. Observe until recovered; otherwise admit.

4. A **seizure** occurs—most minor seizures are very brief and do not require any intervention. If a major tonic–clonic seizure, ensure airway (turn patient on side and remove false teeth) and guard patient from hard-edged or cornered objects that could be injurious. Do not restrain or attempt to separate teeth. Give clonazepam, 1–2 mg intravenously, or Diazemuls 10 mg intravenously. If seizure is prolonged (more than 5 minutes) or status (repeated seizures without intervening recovery of consciousness) develops, repeat injection and request immediate medical assistance. Prolonged seizure activity or status is a medical emergency and may lead to hypoxia, hypotension, and hyperthermia, resulting in permanent brain damage.

Related to psychiatric illness
In general, immediate management is the same as it would be for the psychiatric condition were epilepsy not to be present. However, there are exceptions:

- an **acute psychotic illness** in a patient not known to be psychotic is usually post-ictal. Unless relatives are used to dealing with such episodes, it is best to admit.

- **pseudo-seizures**—the clinician may suspect, and even observe, a seizure that appears non-epileptic. It is better to pass these observations on to the GP or specialist who usually treats the patient's epilepsy, rather than comment directly. If in doubt, treat as for epilepsy.

Response to treatment

Commonly prescribed anticonvulsant drugs

- **Carbamazepine, phenytoin, phenobarbitone**, and **primidone** are first-choice anticonvulsants against most seizure types, with the exception of general absence seizures (petit mal). The last two drugs are now rarely prescribed because of their potential as drugs of abuse.
- **Lamotrigine**, a more recent drug, is effective against a wide range of seizure types including generalized absence seizures.
- **Sodium valproate** is a first choice in primary generalized epilepsy, less so in partial epilepsy.
- **Ethosuximide** is a first-choice drug against generalized absence seizures.
- **Clonazepam** is a first-choice drug against myoclonic and atypical generalized absence seizures.
- **Clobazam, gabapentin**, and **vigabatrin** are second-choice anticonvulsants against partial and secondary generalized seizures.

Careful monitoring of anticonvulsant blood levels is essential, especially at times of change in drug regimen.

Some patients with intractable epilepsy may be eligible for brain surgery.

Course

In most patients (approximately 80%) seizures will be effectively controlled by the first anticonvulsant prescribed. In patients with additional neurological and neuropsychiatric disabilities, control may not be so readily achieved and polytherapy may be unavoidable. Partial seizures are more difficult to control than primary generalized seizures.

Generalized absence seizures usually resolve by the third decade.

Seizures developing for the first time in mid or late life may be associated with progressive underlying pathology and should be investigated with particular care.

Investigations

The investigation of newly suspected epileptic seizures include electroencephalography (EEG) and, particularly in the case of partial seizures, a search for a primary cause. This would include brain imaging (CT, MRI) and routine haematological and biochemical tests. A waking scalp EEG will show relevant abnormalities in only about 50% of cases; a sleep EEG is often more informative. In the case of epilepsy of late onset, periodic re-scanning may be desirable.

When, on clinical grounds, there is considerable doubt about the epileptic nature of the seizures and routine EEG remains negative, a prolonged EEG (telemetry)/video recording may capture a seizure and confirm or refute the diagnosis. In most centres this investigation is carried out over a 5-day period while the patient is in hospital. Seizures must occur with sufficient frequency for this to be an effective investigation.

Patients considered for surgery may undergo tests that assist in localization. These may include telemetry with special electrode placement (foramen ovale, subdural, intracerebral), specialized MRI procedures (volumetric hippocampal measurements, proton spectroscopy), detailed neuropsychological assessment, carotid amytal measurements to determine cerebral dominance and lateralization of memory function, and measures of cerebral blood flow (SPECT, PET) to identify any filling defect.

Head injury

Behavioural and psychosocial problems following head injury are numerous and influential. The Glasgow Coma Scale, duration of coma, and degree of post-traumatic amnesia (PTA) predict the severity of the head injury. A PTA of 24 hours is seen as a watershed: below this, full recovery can be expected; above this, some degree of cognitive impairment is expected. With a PTA of 4 weeks or more, a closed head injury is likely to be followed by invalidism extending over the greater part of a year.

Distinguish between open and closed injuries, the former carrying a higher risk of epilepsy. Contusions occur typically after closed head injury, where the acceleration/deceleration forces and shearing forces lead to damage from localized small vessel bleeding or local destruction. Scattered intracerebral haemorrhages are also found at the interface between grey and white matter. Medial orbital frontal and temporal pole surfaces are key vulnerable areas. Diffuse axonal injury ('diffuse white matter damage') must be considered. This occurs in white matter tracts of the cerebral hemispheres, including the corpus callosum (leading to atrophy and diffuse ventricular enlargement), and the brainstem, particularly the cerebellar peduncles. Over the first 24–48 hours axons break up, forming 'retraction balls'. Clinical findings depend on the severity and extent of brain damage, and include: prolonged coma in the absence of a focal brain lesion; severe cognitive impairment and personality change; and neurological signs, particularly from involvement of long tracts in the brainstem and cerebellar peduncles.

A severe head injury leads to emotional and behavioural problems in about 70% of cases, and these tend to manifest in the year after injury. Impaired self-control and impulsivity, as well as increased dependency and apathy, are evident. There is difficulty in learning from experience, even when new information is retained. Post-traumatic neurotic disorders, particularly anxiety and dysphoria, are seen. Psychosis can occur, with delusions of misidentification observed early in the course of recovery, often associated with more generalized disturbances of insight, judgement, and disorientation.

Early-onset dementias

Creutzfeld–Jakob disease (CJD)

This is a rare, progressive dementia transmitted by infection with a prion (slow virus particle). Spongiform encephalopathy develops, possibly after a prodrome of anxiety or depression. Intellectual decline is followed by spasticity, ataxia, and myoclonic jerks. The terminal stage is of muteness and rigidity, with death occurring within 2 years. EEG may show a characteristic triphasic pattern. Treatment is palliative.

Pick's disease

This rare, probably hereditary, dementia classically affects the frontal lobes initially, but pathology also shows knife-blade atrophy in the temporal lobes. Women are affected more often than men. Presentation is usually between 50 and 60 years of age. Early symptoms are of personality change and selective speech disorder, and later other 'frontal' features as well as memory impairment may be found. Neuroimaging (MRI) reveals frontal, and sometimes anterior, temporal atrophy. Treatment includes genetic counselling.

Huntington's disease

This is an autosomal dominant disorder (triple repeat on short arm chromosome 4). Presentation is usually in the fourth decade of life, with the same incidence in men and women. There is an insidious onset of involuntary choreiform movements affecting the face, head, and arms; initially these can be disguised by the patient. Depression or explosive outbursts may occur. Later, a progressive dementia and athetoid movements are evident. The duration of the disease is 12–16 years. Results of investigation include a 'flat' EEG and caudate atrophy on MRI. Early disease may be detected by looking for decreased metabolism in the caudate with functional neuroimaging. Treatment is low-dose haloperidol or tetrabenazine.

Parkinson's disease

The mean age of onset in this familial disorder is 55 years. Cogwheel rigidity, festinant gait, and bradykinesia are well known, but psychiatric features such as depression are very common. Also, anti-parkinsonian drugs are linked to a variety of psychiatric side-effects, especially psychotic and hallucinatory disorders. In the older patient, arteriosclerotic parkinsonism is frequent, and cognitive impairment here is recognized and associated with the concentration of Lewy bodies. Management should involve liaison with a neurologist.

Normal pressure (communicating) hydrocephalus

Onset is often in later life, but this dementia is potentially reversible. Gait ataxia, cognitive impairment, urinary incontinence, and nystagmus are the clinical features. CSF pressure is normal most of the time, but imaging can reveal enlarged ventricles and cortical atrophy. Treatment is a ventriculoperitoneal shunt.

Amnesic (Korsakoff's) syndrome

This is due to thiamine deficiency, CNS poisoning, or hippocampal damage. A retrograde amnesia (failure to recall events before onset of the disorder) and anterograde amnesia (poor memory for events after the onset of the disorder) are present. There is impaired ability to learn and disorientation for time, but immediate recall is often preserved. Confabulation occurs, perhaps as the patient realizes there is a memory void, but is not diagnostic. There is not an overall global cognitive decline. Treatment is for the underlying cause, but total recovery is exceptional.

CNS infections

Human immunodeficiency virus (HIV)

HIV dementia is now thought to be the commonest dementia in young people. Insidious onset with subtle impairment of memory and concentration are observed initially. Apathy and withdrawal, or social disinhibition, also occur. Poor balance, dysarthria, and tremor may be found, but severe global decline and profound psychomotor retardation develop rapidly. Death due to opportunistic infection, aspiration pneumonia, etc. is the outcome within 2 years for 90% of patients. Space-occupying lesions such as lymphoma are well recognized in HIV disease, and require treatment in a specialist unit. Delirium and a paranoid psychosis, as a result of HIV infection, are also reported; these are treated in the usual way. Adjustment disorders, anxiety, compulsive rituals, and depression are amongst the psychiatric sequelae of HIV diagnosis.

Neurosyphilis

Caused by *Treponema pallidum*, this is now a rare form of organic psychosis and dementia. Frontal lobe involvement is common, leading to personality change, and there is a gradual deterioration in memory and intellect. Depression is often a presenting feature. Argyll Robertson pupils (small, irregular, and unreactive) are seen in more than 50% of cases. Later there is a lower limb weakness, resulting in a spastic paralysis. Serum and CSF VDRL and TPHA tests are positive. High-dose penicillin with steroid cover (to avoid the Herxheimer reaction) is the standard treatment.

Cerebrovascular disease

Cerebrovascular accident (or stroke)

Apart from the physical deficits resulting from stroke, depression is an important sequela that may be overlooked and is said to be more common in dominant anterior lesions. Treatment of choice is probably an SSRI antidepressant. Also, ongoing hypertension or thromboembolic disease needs careful treatment, or progressive cognitive impairment may result.

Subdural haematoma

The peak incidence is between 50 and 60 years. Effects are manifest weeks or months after the initial head injury (which may be trivial). First persistent headache and later recurrent fluctuations in the level of consciousness are seen. Declining memory is usually obvious in long-standing cases, and may be accompanied by neurological signs, such as ipsilateral weakness and hyperreflexia. Radioactive brain scanning is diagnostic in 90% of cases, and CT is helpful. Surgical drainage is often indicated.

Subarachnoid haemorrhage

Subarachnoid haemorrhage is involved in some 8% of strokes, and is associated with high psychiatric morbidity. In addition to the early confusional state, personality change and anxiety are common. Difficulty with attention and concentration rather than a decline in intelligence is seen.

Multiple sclerosis

This condition usually develops after childhood but before 50 years of age. Women are twice as likely to be affected as men, and there is sometimes a positive family history. Psychiatric features include persistent fatigue and depression. Cognitive decline occurs late in the disease, perhaps with associated euphoria. MRI shows white matter lesions or plaques, and visual evoked potentials and CSF oligoclonal immunoglobulin G are diagnostic.

When to refer to experts

Specialist services differ widely in different treatment settings, so the following recommendations are merely a guide. Many specialist services welcome informal discussions before a referral is made and where the referrer is in doubt as to the suitability of the patient or the services provided by the specialist team.

Drug problems

Specialist referral is suggested particularly in the following circumstances:

- The patient requests specialist referral
- The patient has features of the dependence syndrome
- The patient has a complicated pattern of poly-drug use
- The patient is pregnant
- There is risky drug-using behaviour such as injecting

Medical referral should be considered in cases of overdose, or if the following complications are suspected: septicaemia, bacterial endocarditis, hepatitis B, tuberculosis, or HIV infection. Do not forget, however, to involve the general practitioner. Many GPs undertake basic substitute prescribing and are able to provide comprehensive care for their drug-using patients.

Alcohol problems

The following are indicators for specialist referral:

- severe dependence
- history of fits
- history of delirium tremens
- severe concurrent physical or mental illness (including cognitive impairment)
- repeated unsuccessful attempts at outpatient detoxification

The following are medical emergencies requiring immediate hospital admission:

- delirium tremens
- Wernicke's encephalopathy

Sexual and relationship problems

Sexual dysfunction and desire disorders

- Referral of the couple is usually preferable, but individuals are accepted.
- Referrals of patients of any age from 16 years upwards can be accepted.
- Heterosexual and homosexual individuals and couples can be treated.
- If a couple is referred, it is preferable for the relationship to be of at least a few months' duration.
- Patient (and partner) needs to be well motivated for sex therapy.
- Problems of desire, arousal (erection or penetration), and orgasm/ejaculation are appropriate for referral.
- It is better to deal with side-effects of drugs (e.g. antidepressants or antipsychotics) before deciding to refer, as this can sometimes obviate the need for referral.
- The presence of organic factors such as diabetes or multiple sclerosis is not a contraindication to referral; neither is the presence of depression, anxiety, or psychosis.

Sexual, marital and couple therapy

- Be alert to sexual side-effects of drugs.
- Both partners should be referred if in a stable relationship.
- The consent of both partners should be obtained prior to referral.
- The presence of organic causes of sexual dysfunction is not a contraindication to referral.

- Referral to the forensic team may be more appropriate for patients with potentially harmful sexual deviations.

Eating disorders

Effective help is best provided by staff who understand eating disorders. Therefore, referral when the diagnosis is made is preferable. People with eating disorders find that being treated by someone who does not understand the condition is ineffective and may make the condition worse.

Consider emergency admission to a specialized unit for eating disorders or medical ward when the following are present:

- Body mass index is less than $13.5\,\mathrm{kg/m^2}$, especially if more than 25% of body weight is lost in less than 6 months.
- Proximal myopathy.
- Signs of circulatory failure (pulse < 45 per min; blood pressure $< 70/60\,\mathrm{mmHg}$; pregangrenous peripheries, frequent faints).
- Signs of marrow failure (e.g. petechial haemorrhage).
- Severe electrolyte imbalance (e.g. potassium level $< 2.5\,\mathrm{mmol/L}$).
- Hypoglycaemia.

Forensic patients

Forensic psychiatry overlaps with all other psychiatric specialties. All general psychiatrists, for example, will have a significant proportion of individuals with criminal records and antisocial behavioural problems in their case-load. From time to time medicolegal reports will be requested on general psychiatric cases. Forensic psychiatrists do not aim to take on the totality of work concerned with difficult patients and medicolegal issues, but have access to special treatment services, such as maximum security hospitals, medium security units, and prison units. Forensic psychiatrists are also fairly used to managing serious behavioural problems, particularly those that present long-term difficulties. They may, therefore, actively assist in the treatment of cases within the community. Sometimes this is done by the forensic team taking over the care of a difficult patient; sometimes it is done by joint working with regular advice being provided to the core workers.

Advice about management, legal problems, services, and such like can also be sought from forensic psychiatrists without a direct patient referral. Advice may be sought particularly for the following:

- Assessment of dangerousness, especially in the presence of multiple risk factors (see pp. 101–2)
- Assessment of mental state at the time of an offence
- Management of dangerous behaviour
- Advice regarding preparation of medicolegal reports
- Advice on availability and suitability of services

- Referrals to specialist treatment services, such as maximum security hospitals, medium secure units, prison units, and forensic outreach teams
- Technical legal questions.

Neuropsychiatric problems

Specialist neuropsychiatric units usually have a role in the assessment and treatment of the following:
- Psychiatric sequelae of head injury, including depression, cognitive deficits, dementia, and specific lobe syndromes
- Neurological disorders, including Parkinson's disease, Huntington's disease, and motor neuron disorders
- Multisystem disorders, such as systemic lupus erythematosus
- Prion disorders
- Early-onset dementias, including AIDS dementia
- Sleep disorders
- Epilepsy—refer if epilepsy interacts with a psychiatric disorder, or if pseudo-seizures are suspected.

Learning disability

- Always refer when in doubt.
- Refer before commencing any long-term drug therapy, particularly neuroleptics.
- Refer to access community support services. Do not refer simply as a means of disposal.

The elderly

- Many old-age psychiatry services have an age cut-off (e.g. 65 years), but this should not always be followed rigidly.
- Most services will take over the care of patients with presenile dementia (onset before age 65 years).
- Many elderly patients with long-standing functional illness are best managed by the general adult psychiatry team unless they present with new symptoms, such as dementia.

Specialized psychotherapy

All patients referred to a psychiatrist should receive psychological consideration, even if the primary treatment is medication. Selected patients can be referred onwards for specialist assessment and treatment, which, in the NHS, usually means psychodynamic, cognitive behavioural, or systemic (family or couple) therapy. Where referral for specialist psychotherapy is not appropriate, psychotherapists can still contribute to case discussion. The main criteria for patient referral are: someone (a) who is motivated to understand their difficulties in psychological terms and (b) who can contain their anxiety without behaving in unmanageably destructive ways.

Psychodynamic psychotherapy

In thinking about who might benefit from this kind of therapy, diagnosis is less important than personal characteristics. Thus, someone who wishes to address their problems in the context of a relationship, who is not aiming for immediate symptom relief, and who can tolerate the relatively unstructured setting necessary for the optimal exploration of personal difficulties might benefit from this approach. There are no absolute contraindications but, in practice, active drug or alcohol misuse, active psychosis, or a significant tendency towards self-harm or violence would preclude treatment in standard NHS facilities. Most people treated have neurotic or personality problems (e.g. depression, anxiety, difficulties with partners, friends or peers, problems with loss and interdependence), which they inevitably reproduce with the therapist, allowing them to be worked with in a live way. Both individual and group treatments are usually available, the choice depending on a balance of factors including patient preference.

Cognitive behavioural therapy (CBT)

The premise behind this therapy is that thoughts, actions, emotions, and physiology influence one another in a cyclical fashion, and that intervening at any point of the cycle can productively disrupt it. Thus depression is characterized by a negative thought pattern about self, the world, and the future, and may be treated by challenging these thoughts, as well as physiologically (by medication) or behaviourally (by a programme of activity). In cognitive therapy the emphasis is on challenging dysfunctional thinking, although in practice most programmes include a behavioural component. The main criteria for suitability are that the model makes sense to the patient, and that he or she is willing to experiment with alternative ways of thinking, both in the sessions and between them—as 'homework'.

As with other forms of therapy, the patient has to be able to contain anxiety sufficiently to work within the model. However, the more structured nature of the sessions and their more conscious content render CBT inherently less anxiety provoking than psychodynamic therapy. CBT has been shown to be effective in depression, anxiety, phobias, obsessional compulsive and eating disorders, among others. In addition, some aspects of psychosis are amenable to CBT and, less commonly, the techniques have been used in groups. People with personality disorders may respond to longer-term, more specialized, CBT, although psychodynamic therapy is often the preferred option in these cases.

Family therapy

Unlike most other therapies, useful work can be done in the sessions even when the index patient is too ill to participate fully. This is because resultant shifts in the family system may operate to the patient's (as well as to the family's) benefit. Moreover, the iller the patient, the more the family is entitled to consideration in its own right, especially as family members may be involved in long-term care and support. A great deal can be gained by making a family dynamic assessment early on in treatment and, in principle, any family whose members expresses a willingness to work together with a skilled professional to help their ill member is suitable for referral for family therapy. Family therapy has been shown to be effective in reducing relapse in schizophrenia, as well as in adolescent anorexia nervosa, and as a couple treatment for depression where one partner is affected. In family therapy no clear distinction is made between assessment and therapy: the first session aims to establish a treatment contract and this contract is reviewed regularly. In practice, a typical contract might involve four to six sessions over a 2–3-month period, depending on response.

Case discussion

Psychotherapists can offer discussion of complicated cases, even when these are unlikely to be suitable for psychotherapy. This can happen as a one-off, or as part of a regular seminar attended by all members of the multidisciplinary team. In practice, these seminars tend to be offered by psychodynamically oriented therapists, who are trained to think about the dynamics evoked in the team as well as about the individual patient. The patients discussed tend to be those who generate most emotion and controversy among those trying to help them, and who often suffer from a personality disorder in addition to the 'Axis I' diagnosis. Case discussions help the staff to keep track of countertransference interference with sound judgement and good management.

Early treatments

Acute psychosis

Advice on rapid tranquillization is given in Fig. 10.1. Appendix 4 contains a list of antipsychotic drugs and Appendix 5 gives long-acting preparations. Equivalent doses of various neuroleptics are given in Appendix 6, and information about clozapine in Appendix 7.

Management of acute psychosis

A patient with a first episode of schizophrenic psychosis should receive either an atypical antipsychotic or a low-dose typical antipsychotic for at least 6 weeks. Many believe that atypicals are better tolerated than typical drugs; certainly, they induce fewer extrapyramidal side-effects at normal doses. In case of failure of the first treatment, it is important to review compliance and tolerability. If the patient

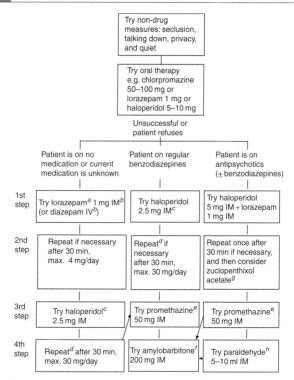

Figure 10.1 Algorithm for the management of acute disturbed or violent behaviour (modified after droperidol was withdrawn in the UK).

shows poor or no response, despite full compliance, it is better to switch to another drug and to assess over another 6 weeks.

When a patient with a previous history of schizophrenia experiences a relapse, the adherence to treatment should be assessed thoroughly, as well as the possible social and psychological precipitants. If full adherence to medication is confirmed, the usual drug treatment may be continued (in combination with a short-term sedative, if required in the acute phase). Alternatively, one can consider switching to a different antipsychotic (and assess over the following 6 weeks). If this second antipsychotic treatment proves ineffective, then clozapine should be considered as the next alternative. When adherence to treatment is poor, it is important to investigate the reasons. Compliance aids and education may be helpful. If the poor compliance is related to poor tolerability, the use of a different drug should be discussed with the patient. Treatment with a depot preparation may be necessary.

Acute dystonia affecting respiration

Clinical features

Abrupt onset, hours after commencing neuroleptic (often butyrophenone). Young people are affected more than older ones. Involves painful muscular spasm with respiratory stridor and tongue protrusion, which induces panic.

Differential diagnosis

Status epilepticus; trismus; foreign body obstruction; hysteria (rare).

Management

Stop the neuroleptic. Give intramuscular procyclidine 5–10 mg or equivalent. Reassure patient and staff. Check for cyanosis and administer oxygen; transfer to medical unit as required.

Neuroleptic malignant syndrome

Neuroleptic malignant syndrome (NMS) is a rare idiosyncratic reaction to neuroleptics characterized by:

* intense extrapyramidal rigidity and other dystonia
* pyrexia, which may be mild
* autonomic dysfunction
* diaphoresis
* clouding of consciousness.

There is substantial overlap with acute lethal catatonia. The incidence of the condition is variously reported as between 0.07% and 2%, probably because of the lack of clear diagnostic criteria and the overlap with other severe extrapyramidal syndromes. Associated biochemical and other abnormalities include a grossly raised level of **creatine phosphokinase, leucocytosis**, and a **raised ESR**.

NMS has been reported with all neuroleptics and is unpredictable, although it tends to be associated with larger doses of high-potency antipsychotics. Its reported mortality rate varies between 12% and 18%, usually as a consequence of autonomic instability (e.g. cardiac arrest) or renal failure due to rhabdomyolysis and myoglobinuria.

Treatment of neuroleptic malignant syndrome

Ideally, all patients suspected of having NMS should be transferred to a medical intensive care facility. Immediate withdrawal of neuroleptics usually produces rapid resolution in patients identified early. A dopamine agonist such as oral **bromocriptine** or subcutaneous **apomorphine** is also recommended, and sometimes **dantrolene** as a peripheral skeletal muscle relaxant can be given intravenously up to five times. Full medical supportive measures to maintain hydration, electrolyte status and renal function should be available. In established cases, these measures should lead to a resolution over about 10 days.

An algorithm for the treatment of NMS is given in Fig. 10.2.

Treatment of the remaining psychiatric problems

If the patient's psychiatric condition still demands treatment, **ECT** would appear to be the safest option. However, this should be deferred until after the episode as the anaesthetic risk is increased with autonomic dysfunction. A 'drug holiday' of 2 weeks is certainly recommended and diminishes the chance of recurrence on re-challenge. Re-challenge is best with a lower-potency neuroleptic of a different chemical class. Patients need daily physical monitoring of blood pressure, consciousness,

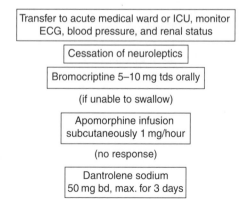

Figure 10.2 Algorithm for the treatment of neuroleptic malignant syndrome.

and temperature, and creatinine phosphokinase (CPK) estimations during re-challenge. About one in six patients will suffer a recurrence after a re-challenge.

Acute mania and catatonia

Acute manic episodes are best treated with a mood stabilizer: lithium (target plasma concentration 0.6–1.2 mmol/L), carbamazepine (target plasma concentration 8–12 mg/L), or sodium valproate (target plasma concentration 50–100 mg/L). Sedation in response to the behavioural disturbance will require benzodiazepine (lorazepam 1 mg tds or clonazepam 1 mg bd), to be assessed over 2–3 days and withdrawn following the resolution of symptoms. If the mood stabilizers (with or without the benzodiazepines) are ineffective, start an antipsychotic (haloperidol 5 mg t.d.s., chlorpromazine 100 mg t.d.s., or olanzapine 10 mg/day). Antipsychotics may be considered at an earlier stage if psychotic symptoms are present. Evaluate the response to the antipsychotics over 1–2 weeks and withdraw after resolution of symptoms.

In severely disturbed patients or patients refusing medication or in a manic emergency, ECT may occasionally be considered. This should be bilateral because of the need for a rapid response. The disturbance usually abates after one or two applications.

Catatonia is rarely seen in developed countries now. The most important principle in treating catatonia is to distinguish it from NMS and manic or depressive stupor (see p. 83). Catatonia, in acute schizophrenia, may be characterized by waxy flexibility, negativism, automatic obedience, and a 'wooden' affect. Treatment of the catatonia is of the underlying condition. However, in persistent or distressing states, benzodiazepines or ECT may be tried.

Severe depression

Antidepressant treatment

Antidepressants are the mainstay of treatment. Their effectiveness should be assessed 4–6 weeks after reaching the therapeutic dose. In case of poor tolerability or inadequate response to the maximum tolerable dose, switch to a different antidepressant. When switching between antidepressants, abrupt withdrawal should be avoided and cross-tapering should be used. All antidepressants have the potential to cause withdrawal phenomena when stopped abruptly; therefore, antidepressants should always be withdrawn slowly, preferably over 4 weeks. Common symptoms of antidepressant discontinuation are: dizziness, electric shock sensations, anxiety and agitation, insomnia, flu-like symptoms, diarrhoea and abdominal spasms, paraesthesia, mood swings, nausea, and low mood. If withdrawal symptoms occur, slow the rate of drug withdrawal and return to the last dose tolerated by the patient. If the drug has been stopped, give reassurance: symptoms rarely last for more than 1–2 weeks.

Levels of inpatient supervision for a suicidal patient

When a suicidal patient is admitted, the admitting doctor should discuss the level of supervision with a senior nurse. The options are:

1. **Close observation:** Here the patient is always in sight of the supervising nurse. This is normal practice when a depressed patient with a high suicide risk is admitted. Usually the risk abates within a few days, but the level of risk needs to be assessed daily.

2. **Continuous supervision:** Here the patient is always within reach of a nurse. This is used when the patient is at immediate risk from self-destructive, including bulimic, behaviour.

3. **Routine nursing care.**

Assessment of other physical risk

Weight loss is common and, unless severe, is not a cause for concern, but dehydration is always an indication for admission and institution of a fluid balance chart with assessment of electrolyte levels. Skilled nursing persuades many patients to drink, but if this fails then other action is needed, including—very occasionally—intravenous rehydration and emergency ECT.

Prescribing in pregnancy and breast-feeding

Drugs with which there has been the most experience are generally preferred in pregnancy. Tricyclics are the antidepressants of choice, especially nortriptyline, amitriptyline, and imipramine. Of the SSRIs, fluoxetine is not thought to be associated with obstetric complications or fetal malformations. Chlorpromazine and trifluoperazine are the antipsychotics of choice. Depot preparations and atypical antipsychotics are best avoided. When a sedative is necessary, promethazine can be used. The mood stabilizers—lithium, carbamazepine, and sodium valproate—are all best avoided during the first trimester.

Few systematic studies have been performed on the use of psychotropic drugs during breast-feeding. If the mother is taking psychotropic drugs, breast-feeding should certainly be avoided if the infant has evidence of impaired renal, liver, cardiovascular, or neurological functions. Breast-feeding should also be avoided when the mother is taking MAOIs, lithium, or clozapine. Tricyclics (not doxepine) seem to be safe. Fewer data have been published on SSRIs, although initial evidence suggests only minor effects on infants. Among antipsychotics, chlorpromazine, haloperidol, and trifluoperazine can be used, if the doses are not increased. Valproate and carbamazepine seem relatively safe.

Electroconvulsive therapy

Advances in pharmacological and psychological treatments have meant that ECT is needed much less frequently than formerly.

The editors' view is that it should be used only when absolutely necessary. Many patients (and their relatives) are afraid of it, and great care should be taken in explaining the procedure, the aim of treatment, and side-effects to them; written information should also be made available. One should be very cautious about compulsory ECT, but where this is unavoidable the relevant legal powers to administer it will need to be invoked before the treatment.

Detailed information about ECT can be found in "The ECT Handbook", the Second Report of the Royal College of Psychiatrists' Special Committee on ECT. The Royal College has produced a training video, with the aim of updating and improving standards of ECT administration. Your individual hospital may have a local policy or guidelines relating to the administration of ECT with which you should be familiar. You should also be familiar with the relevant mental health legislation.

Indications

Depressive illnesses

ECT is an effective treatment for severe depression but is necessary only in a small proportion of depressed patients. It is particularly useful when symptoms include psychomotor retardation and psychotic features such as delusions and/or hallucinations. It can be life-saving if the patient is very acutely suicidal or in the rare instance where the patient fails to maintain an adequate nutritional or hydration status. Other indications for its use include patient preference, a past history of response to ECT, the need for a rapid response to treatment, and when the risks of other treatments exceed those of ECT. Old-age psychiatrists may recommend its use in the depressed elderly who have not responded to drug treatments or who have suffered unpleasant side-effects.

Manic illness

ECT is infrequently used for mania. Indications for its use include the need for a speedy therapeutic response, as a safe alternative to high-dose medications, or if patients have drug-resistant mania or 'rapid cycling' mania.

Schizophrenia

There are few indications for ECT in schizophrenia in Western societies. Very occasionally it may be used when psychotic symptoms are associated with abnormal motor activity such as catatonic excitement or immobility. It may be considered if the patient is unable to tolerate medications or has failed to respond to an adequate dose of antipsychotics, including clozapine.

Other conditions

ECT can occasionally be useful in the postpartum psychoses, the neuroleptic malignant syndrome, and catatonia. It has also been used occasionally in severe delirium, resistant epilepsy, and Parkinson's disease (particularly those with the 'on–off' phenomenon).

Contraindications

Although there are no absolute contraindications to ECT, coexisting medical illnesses must be treated. Close liaison between the psychiatrist, anaesthetist, and physicians may be necessary. Pregnancy and old age are not contraindications to ECT, but ECT involves an anaesthetic and any contraindications to anaesthesia will apply; 'high-risk' patients with recent myocardial infarction, stroke, or raised intracranial pressure should be assessed on an individual basis in consultation with the anaesthetist. Those with known cardiac disease will need assessment by a physician or cardiologist prior to ECT. ECG monitoring may be necessary during ECT administration, and the need for staff adequately trained in cardiopulmonary resuscitation and management of arrhythmias should be recognized. Following myocardial infarction, ECT should be delayed as long as possible, and is probably safer after 3 months.

Side-effects

The mortality rate associated with ECT is approximately 2 per 100 000 treatments, a figure similar to that for minor surgical procedures. The most common side-effects include headache, memory impairment, and confusion. Rarer side-effects include prolonged seizures, tardive seizures, manic rebound, and physical complications such as ruptured bladder or aspiration pneumonia. Modification of anaesthesia with a barbiturate anaesthetic and muscle relaxant have decreased morbidity, as have improvements in ECT monitoring. While bilateral application of ECT is the recommended means of inducing a seizure, the use of unilateral non-dominant ECT can be used if cognitive side-effects are troublesome.

Preparation

A full physical examination and history are required for every patient. In addition to baseline blood tests for electrolytes and full blood count, the need for other tests such as a sickle cell screen should be considered. ECG and chest radiography will be needed if there is a history of cardiac disease or other physical illnesses, and the anaesthetist should be notified of any significant physical illnesses.

Patients should be fasted for at least 6 hours before the procedure, as with all general anaesthetics. As benzodiazepines are powerful anticonvulsants, acute dosing should be avoided immediately before ECT, and even short-acting benzodiazepines may be present in significant quantities the morning after their use for night sedation. However, patients who are chronic benzodiazepine users have a lower threshold for seizure during benzodiazepine withdrawal and abrupt reductions in dosage are best avoided during ECT. Similarly anticonvulsants raise the seizure threshold and higher stimulus energies may be needed for treatment. If anticonvulsants are needed to control epilepsy, their effect should be to return seizure threshold to normal. If prescribed for mood stabilization, it may be best to continue them during ECT. Neuroleptics tend to be proconvulsant.

Inpatients should be accompanied to the ECT suite by a member of staff whom they trust. Ward staff should have completed a pre-ECT checklist, detailing general observations including removal of jewellery and dentures as appropriate. You should have access to the case notes and the current and past drug prescription chart; also, the consultant's prescription for ECT, which documents the indications for ECT, relevant past medical history, past treatments, legal status, and past psychiatric history, should be available. If the patient has previously had ECT, then previous prescription charts can give useful information about previous stimulus energy required. Fully informed consent must be obtained and documented, or the relevant legal documents pertinent to the administration of ECT must be available for scrutiny.

Administration

The procedures must be carried out meticulously. The ECT machine should be safe and easy to use. You should be familiar with the machine, and must have received detailed and appropriate instructions in its use from a senior clinician. EEG monitoring is desirable. Electrode placement can be either bilateral or unilateral; bilateral placement is routinely used. Unilateral placement is associated with substantially less memory impairment than bilateral placement; however, bilateral ECT is preferable where a rapid response is required. Local policy may dictate the use of stimulus titration and the initial dosage given. There is a 40-fold difference in seizure threshold between individuals, and ECT is itself anticonvulsant, raising the seizure threshold during a course of treatment.

A therapeutic seizure should be bilateral and of approximately 15 seconds' duration visually and 20–50 seconds on EEG (if available). Prolonged seizures are those that last for 2 minutes or more, and should be terminated immediately either with further induction agent or with intravenous diazepam. The number of treatments will be determined by clinical progress. Stimulus dosages at follow-up treatments may be estimated from the previous stimulus dose used (allowing for the increase in seizure threshold caused by ECT). A common policy is twice-weekly administration for 6 to 12 treatments.

Deliberate self-harm

Assess the patient's mental state in the light of the social environment and coping skills (see pp. 27–9):

1. Treatment of the physical condition of patients with deliberate self-harm (DSH) takes precedence (remember the liver toxicity of paracetamol).

2. Suicide and risk of repetition cannot be assessed in a drowsy patient.

3. In patients with low repetition risk and no mental illness, the principles of **crisis intervention** apply: 'understand' the attempt, mobilize resources, consider a 'non-DSH' contract, discharge preferably to relatives, inform GP, appointment with DSH-liaison or alcohol/drugs services team.

4. High-risk patients—most are mentally ill. Management depends on the community resources available (e.g. supportive relatives, GP, CPN). In case of unacceptable risk, consider admission, compulsorily if necessary.

5. Frequent repeaters—the same principles apply; a long-term management plan is vital to avoid counterproductive admissions.

6. Risk can never be excluded completely; careful note-taking and interdisciplinary communication are vital for your patient's health and your own protection.

Opiate overdose causes varying degrees of coma, respiratory depression, and pinpoint pupils. The short-acting opiate antagonist naloxone is indicated if there is coma or bradypnoea. The dosage is 0.8–2 mg, repeated at intervals of 2–3 minutes to a maximum of 10 mg if respiratory function does not improve. Naloxone is available in preloaded syringes. Owing to its short action, it may be necessary to set up a naloxone infusion, which is adjusted according to response. This may occur in patients who have overdosed on methadone because it has a long half-life. In severe cases, mechanical ventilation may be necessary.

Following the administration of naloxone, a patient will experience acute withdrawal. It is important to continue to observe them for 24 hours, but commonly craving for drugs will lead them to discharge themselves.

If **methadone overdose** is reported but there are not yet any signs of respiratory depression, activated charcoal should be given and the patient observed closely. Inducing patients to vomit is not recommended because of the risk of rapid onset of CNS depression and unconsciousness, which could lead to choking.

Cocaine overdose is characterized by cardiovascular complications including arrhythmias, cardiac ischaemia, myocarditis, cardiomyopathy, and hypertension. Seizures and hyperpyrexia also occur. Treatment is supportive and patients need medical help as soon as possible.

Alcohol dependence

Alcohol withdrawal syndrome

Individuals will experience symptoms of alcohol withdrawal only if they are physically dependent on alcohol. Thus, some heavy drinkers experience no withdrawal symptoms, whereas others show evidence of mild or moderate withdrawal, and a few will develop a life-threatening disturbance.

Symptoms of alcohol withdrawal start approximately 3–6 hours after the last drink. Early symptoms include tremor, sweats, nausea, insomnia, and anxiety. Transient auditory hallucinations in clear consciousness may occur. There is a risk of alcohol withdrawal seizures at between 10 and 60 hours; these generalized (grand mal) seizures are often associated with hypoglycaemia, hypokalaemia, hypomagnesaemia, and concurrent epilepsy. Most alcohol withdrawal syndromes resolve within 72 hours of drinking cessation. The more severe the withdrawal, the longer the duration. A few patients go on to develop delirium tremens (DTs) about 72 hours after the last drink. Symptoms include severe clouding of consciousness, confusion, hallucinations in any modality, tremor, fear, paranoid delusions, restlessness, and agitation. The condition usually lasts for 3–5 days, with gradual resolution. Predisposing factors include hypoglycaemia, hypokalaemia, hypocalcaemia, and intercurrent infection.

Delirium tremens and Wernicke's encephalopathy are medical emergencies requiring immediate hospital admission.

Treatment of alcohol withdrawal

Most patients can be detoxified safely and effectively in the community. Indications for inpatient detoxification include severe dependence, a history of delirium tremens or alcohol withdrawal seizures, coexistent medical problems, an unsupportive home environment, and a previously failed community detoxification. All patients need general support and a proportion will need pharmacotherapy for the withdrawal symptoms. Benzodiazepines are the treatment of choice and individual doctors should become familiar with one drug of this class. Because of the great range in the severity of the alcohol withdrawal syndrome, a range of drug doses is indicated. A mild to moderate withdrawal syndrome in an outpatient should respond to chlordiazepoxide (Librium) 5–10 mg three or four times daily. A moderate withdrawal syndrome may require a dose in the order of 15–20 mg three or four times daily. Community and out patient detoxifications should last approximately 1 week. In an inpatient setting, the chlordiazepoxide is prescribed according to a flexible regimen over the first 24 hours, with dosage titrated against the severity of withdrawal symptoms. Higher doses are usually required in the inpatient setting, for example chlordiazepoxide 40–60 mg three or four times a day, reducing over 5 days. However, a longer regimen may be required in the case of patients who have delirium tremens or a history of delirium tremens.

Chlormethiazole (Heminevrin) still has a role in the inpatient setting but is contraindicated for community detoxification because of its potential for dependence.

Appropriate treatment as above should prevent the development of alcohol withdrawal seizures, and anticonvulsants are not indicated routinely. However, carbamazepine may be considered if there is a history of seizures during any previous withdrawal episodes, or a history of untreated epilepsy.

Because of the risk of Wernicke's encephalopathy in these patients, prophylactic thiamine (vitamin B) supplementation is recommended. Thiamine may be taken orally, but absorption is poor. Prophylactic treatment for Wernicke's encephalopathy should be one pair of intramuscular (IM) or intravenous (IV) ampoules of high-potency B-complex vitamins (Pabrinex) daily for 3–5 days (or thiamine 200–300 mg intramuscularly daily, if Pabrinex is not available). Parenteral vitamin supplements should be administered only if suitable resuscitation facilities are immediately available.

Delirium tremens

Clinical features

Alcohol withdrawal phenomena. Rapid onset of hallucinations, fear, disorientation and confusion, tremor, tachycardia, fever, overactivity, and clamminess (not always the full house!).

Differential diagnosis

Delirium due to another cause.

Management

The full-blown syndrome should be managed on a medical unit (mortality rate greater than 5%). Give adequate sedation (chlordiazepoxide 40 mg qds) and fluid replacement. Administer vitamins (thiamine) as a prophylactic. Beware withdrawal seizures.

Wernicke's encephalopathy

Clinical features

The classical picture is of acute onset of nystagmus, gaze palsies, gait ataxia, and confusional state due to thiamine deficiency, but not all patients show the full picture. Wernicke's encephalopathy is most commonly seen in alcoholics, but may also occur in malnutrition and prolonged vomiting (including in eating disorders).

Differential diagnosis

This includes infective or metabolic encephalopathy, hydrocephalus, tumour, posterior circulation infarction, or haemorrhage.

Management

Treatment should be given as soon as the diagnosis is entertained, preferably intravenously. This should be at least two pairs of IM or IV ampoules of high-potency B-complex vitamins daily for 2 days. If symptoms respond, continue with one pair of ampoules daily for 5 days or as long as improvement continues.

Drug misuse

Basic management

- Knowledge of local patterns of drug use, practicalities of drug use, and terms used can be important in establishing rapport.

- A non-judgemental attitude both with regard to drug use and associated activity such as sex work is essential.

- Consistency of communication between different staff members is important to minimize the potential for confused messages.

- Be clear about what the patient can expect in the way of treatment in your particular setting.

- Be clear about what is expected of the patient in your treatment setting.

- Your contact with a drug user may be the only one they have with services for some time, especially if it takes place in an emergency setting. Emphasizing general healthcare needs, education, and harm reduction (see section on this topic) advice is important in this situation.

- Change in drug use in established misusers usually takes place by means of several cycles of contemplation, change, and relapse. Avoid the disappointment that can result from expectation of sudden lasting change, but maintain hope and optimism in your attitude!

Opiates

Opiate withdrawal

Symptoms of withdrawal from heroin can be expected to start within 12 hours of the last dose of the drug. They peak within 72 hours and are likely to be essentially over within a week, although milder symptoms and sleep difficulty may persist for several weeks. Patients met in clinical practice are also likely to be withdrawing from methadone, which has a longer half-life and therefore a withdrawal syndrome that is delayed in onset (usually at least 24 hours after the last dose), peaking after several days and likely to last longer than a week. The pattern of withdrawal from other opiates may be predicted from the half-life and dose. Withdrawal from partial opiate agonists (e.g. buprenorphine) is typically described as milder than that from full agonists.

Withdrawal from opiates is due to unopposed activity by neurotransmitter systems that have adapted to the presence of opiates. The symptoms can be predicted from consideration of the effects of unopposed high levels of activity in the locus coeruleus (central noradrenergic) and peripheral sympathetic autonomic activity:

- pupillary dilatation

- rhinorrhoea

- lacrymation

- sneezing
- piloerection
- nausea
- vomiting
- abdominal cramp
- diarrhoea
- skeletal muscle cramp
- anxiety
- dysphoria
- tachycardia
- raised blood pressure.

Craving for opiates and opiate-seeking behaviour are also likely to be present.

Withdrawal of opiates can reveal masked underlying symptoms such as pain. Although markedly unpleasant, the withdrawal syndrome is not directly physically dangerous. The severity of opiate withdrawal may be expected to vary with the dose of opiate, but is also susceptible to other factors such as the physical and social environment.

Symptomatic relief with non-opiate medication This is an option that can be offered by any doctor when a patient presents in withdrawal. Medications to consider include:

- metaclopramide
- Lomotil
- mebeverine.

These drugs should be prescribed in normal dosage for the duration of the withdrawal period. Diazepam may also be appropriate in this situation to help sleep, muscle spasm, and anxiety. However, it should be prescribed only when there is no suspicion of benzodiazepine mis-use by the patient, in moderate doses, and strictly for the duration of the expected withdrawal period only.

Methadone Methadone is commonly used to assist withdrawal from opiates. Initially the patient should be stabilized on a dose of methadone sufficient to control withdrawal symptoms. The dose of methadone is then tapered according to an exponential decay curve (i.e. larger decrements initially). In practice, the time over which this is done varies with the situation, from reduction over 10 days in inpatient settings to much slower reduction in outpatients. Overall benefit is probably greatest if the reduction regimen proceeds flexibly, as planned with the patient, rather than rigidly according to a protocol.

Lofexidine Lofexidine is a centrally acting α_2 agonist that is licensed for the management of withdrawal symptoms. It has the advantage of causing less hypotension than clonidine (another centrally acting α_2

agonist that has been used for some time in inpatient settings). When prescribing lofexidine, it is important to monitor blood pressure and pulse at baseline and during treatment. Recommended doses are 0.4–0.6 mg twice daily initially, to be increased if necessary to control withdrawal symptoms in steps of 0.2–0.4 mg daily to a maximum total daily dose of 2.4 mg. The total daily dose should be given in two to four divided doses. The treatment course should be 7–10 days, followed by a gradual withdrawal over 2–4 days.

Opiates: basic substitute prescribing

Methadone is a synthetic long-acting opiate that may be taken by mouth. Substitute prescribing of methadone for heroin provides opportunities for several types of treatment, i.e.

- Short-term detoxification
- Longer-term (months) outpatient effort to achieve abstinence
- Maintenance treatment in which the aim does not include abstinence except in the much longer term (years). Treatment aims of maintenance are reduction in frequency of injecting, reduction in the amount of illicit drug use, reduction in crime, social and psychological stabilization (see section on harm reduction).

There are several issues that are common to all methadone prescribing. Before starting, it should be established that the patient is already opiate dependent. Methods include:

- history taking
- detection of heroin in several urine samples
- inspection of injection sites in an intra-venous user
- observation of withdrawal symptoms.

The initial dose of methadone can be estimated from the history of heroin consumption, but it is usual to start with a safe dose (20 mg in adults) administered in a setting where response can be assessed later that day or the following day, and gradually titrating the dose up to the desired dose. In a situation aimed at detoxification, the dose will be the lowest that controls withdrawal symptoms, but may be considerably higher when maintenance is the aim because higher doses are associated with better outcomes.

Methadone is prescribed from a hospital on a pink prescription, which allows for multiple dispensing dates. It should usually be prescribed for dispensing on a daily basis. The prescription needs to contain the type of methadone, daily dose and total amount in words and figures, frequency of dispensing, and start date. For example:

> Methadone mixture 1 mg/mL DTF 40 mg (forty) daily for 14 days. Dispense daily, but for two days on Saturdays. Start on 1st July 1998. Total dose 560 mg (five hundred and sixty)

The conditions on which the prescription is offered should be clearly agreed between the patient and the prescriber before commencing a prescription. Issues to be agreed include length of prescription, frequency with which the prescriber will see the patient, lack of acceptability of aggression, threats or actual violence, alcohol consumption, urine testing in which heroin and methadone use can be distinguished and whether continued evidence of illicit drug use is acceptable, other treatment to be offered in addition to prescribing. It is good practice also to identify, at the outset, the targets that it is anticipated the treatment offered will help the patient to achieve, and future dates at which treatment will be reviewed.

Benzodiazepines

Benzodiazepine withdrawal

The benzodiazepine group of drugs also contains drugs with a wide range of half-lives, which affects the pattern and severity of withdrawal syndrome. Examples are:

Short acting

    triazolam

    temazepam

Intermediate

    oxazepam

    nitrazepam

Long acting

    diazepam

    flunitrazepam

Onset of symptoms may be rapid, as in the case of triazolam, which has been reported to result in rebound wakefulness and withdrawal within the course of a single night (resulting in its withdrawal from the UK market). In clinical practice with the street drug-using population, the most likely benzodiazepines to be encountered are temazepam and diazepam. Often the use will be a mixture including these two. Withdrawal symptoms will have an insidious onset in this situation and may occur days after the last dose of diazepam. Symptoms are due to unopposed activity of the GABA complex. They consist of general symptoms of anxiety:

- tremor
- tachycardia
- tachypnoea
- nausea
- abdominal cramp
- skeletal muscle cramp

- diarrhoea
- psychic anxiety

and in addition:

- seizures
- perceptual distortion.

The symptoms can be more subtle and difficult to distinguish from those of other conditions, such as anxiety disorders, than opiate withdrawal. However, benzodiazepine withdrawal carries a greater physical danger because of the risk of seizures.

Stabilization on to diazepam and gradual tapering of the dose will control withdrawal symptoms. As with opiates, the time over which the tapering occurs is shorter and more rigidly determined in inpatients (10–21 days). Reduction in outpatients is more likely to take place over the course of several weeks and to involve the patient in determining the rate of reduction (see section on substitute prescribing).

In patients with an established history of seizures, a covering dose of an antiepileptic such as carbamazepine may aid a planned detoxification.

Benzodiazepines: basic substitute prescribing

Diazepam is usually chosen as a substitute for illicit diazepam, temazepam, and other benzodiazepines. This is primarily due to its long half-life. The evidence basis for its success in substitute prescribing in the population of drug misusers, who are usually poly-drug misusers, is much more controversial than that of methadone for heroin. There is no obvious benefit in terms of changed injecting practice, for example, in many cases. It is harder to be clear in follow-up whether the patient is being compliant because urine testing provides no useful evidence to back up clinical history and examination. In practice, decisions are made according to local practice, local population of drug misusers, and individual clinical assessment.

A starting dose of diazepam is negotiated that will prevent withdrawal, and a reduction regimen is agreed with the patient before starting the prescription. The agreement may set out a rigid structure or may simply be the boundaries within which change will be negotiated as the treatment progresses. Most benzodiazepine prescribing is done with abstinence as a goal at least within a few months, but there are some individuals for whom a period of maintenance is agreed. Diazepam can currently be prescribed only on yellow single-dispensing prescriptions in the UK. Arranging daily dispensing, although desirable in many cases, is often inconvenient or impossible. As with methadone, agreement of the conditions of treatment, criteria for review, and frequency of review must be clear at the outset.

Amphetamines, cocaine, and other stimulant drugs

Stimulant drugs such as amphetamines, cocaine, and 'ecstasy' do not produce a major physical withdrawal syndrome and can be stopped abruptly. Many stimulant users who are psychologically dependent experience insomnia and depressed mood when the drug is stopped. Antidepressants such as desipramine may be helpful, but many stimulant users just need advice regarding the likely symptoms, reassurance that they will pass, and a safe place to get through this period. Some patients may become acutely suicidal and will require hospital admission and close observation.

Substitute prescribing of stimulant drugs is rarely recommended and should be left for specialist treatment services. However, remember that stimulant drugs, like opiates, may be injected, and advice on harm reduction may be appropriate (see section on harm reduction).

Stimulant-induced confusion and anxiety states

Cocaine and other stimulants such as ecstasy (MDMA) and amphetamines can cause acute effects that can sometimes be severe enough to present to the general psychiatrist. These states are commonly of euphoria or anxiety, but may proceed to more severe symptoms such as paranoid ideation leading to vigilant and aggressive behaviour and auditory or visual hallucinations. Insight is usually retained or only transiently impaired. Management involves calming and reassuring the patient until the effects wear off. Occasionally oral diazepam (10–20 mg) may be needed and in severe cases anti-psychotic medication. If symptoms persist they may become a drug induced psychosis requiring general psychiatric management.

Hallucinogenic drugs

Hallucinogenic drugs such as LSD do not produce a physical withdrawal syndrome and can be stopped abruptly. There is no role for substitute prescribing. However, some people experience severe psychological distress during or after use of hallucinogens and may need symptomatic treatment (such as a brief course of benzodiazepines to reduce anxiety) and a safe place to be while the experience passes.

Harm reduction

This is an approach to the management of drug users that was developed following the discovery of HIV in the intravenous drug-using population. The transmission of blood-borne viruses is one of many possible harms from drug use. The approach assumes that reducing the harm from the use of drugs may take priority over the reduction of drug use itself. It assumes a hierarchy of treatment goals, with abstinence being the ideal outcome but with intermediate goals achievable. For instance, an objective may be to reduce intravenous drug use and transfer to oral drug use or to move from risky injecting where needles are being shared to safer injecting using clean injecting equipment.

Basic harm reduction advice should be available whenever a drug user presents to a service and should include education about the following:

1. Safe injecting techniques, including not sharing or reusing needles, skin cleaning, and advice about the danger of some injecting sites—particularly groin and femoral.

2. Advice on how to obtain clean injecting equipment. This will depend on the area but may be from a local drugs agency or a pharmacy needle exchange scheme.

3. Advice on safer sex. This will include advice on how the virus is transmitted sexually—by vaginal or anal intercourse and less frequently by oral sex—and on the correct use of condoms.

4. Advice on how to clean injecting equipment if it must be reused. This is done using ordinary domestic bleach and at least three rinses with clean cold water.

5. Advice on the dangers of overdose from opiates. This includes an awareness of problems with losing tolerance after a period of lower drug intake, such as in prison, and the dangers of new supplies of drug that may have higher purity.

6. Advice on the dangers of prescribed and non-prescribed drugs to children. Methadone overdoses in children are common and any amount may be dangerous and necessitate hospital treatment.

Other harm reduction interventions for drug users include:

- Hepatitis B immunization for non-immune individuals.
- HIV and hepatitis testing with appropriate counselling before and after testing.
- Prescription of oral substitute drugs (see section on basic substitute prescribing).

Eating disorders

Anorexia nervosa

Outpatient psychotherapy or counselling is effective if there has not been too much weight loss (less than 25%). Specialist psychotherapy such as cognitive analytical therapy or modified dynamic therapy is more effective than supportive psychotherapy. Frequently the therapy has to be continued long term. It is important that this is supplemented by regular medical monitoring. It is helpful to have the family of patients under the age of 17 years involved in treatment. Parental counselling is as effective and more acceptable to the family than family therapy.

Inpatient treatment is necessary for those with severe weight loss. Staff with expertise in the management of eating disorders can provide a judicious mixture of psychotherapy and nutritional support. In extreme circumstances people may be detained under the Mental Health Act.

Bulimia nervosa

The Royal College of Psychiatrist's Report recommends a stepped approach to treatment. Low-intensity interventions such as self-help manuals, groups, or guided self-care are useful in the first instance. Medium-term interventions such as cognitive behavioural or interpersonal therapy require more specialist skills. Patients with personality difficulties, for example the multi-impulsive or borderline patient or those with additional physical morbidity such as diabetes mellitus, may need long-term psychotherapy or inpatient treatment.

Treatment must address the psychological aspects of anorexia and bulimia nervosa as well as the eating behaviour. Re-feeding alone may be successful in short-term weight restoration, but is usually not effective in the long term.

Investigations recommended for eating disorders on initial assessment

- Full blood count (cells reduced: WCC > RBC > platelets).
- Urea and electrolytes (low potassium, magnesium, calcium, and phosphate levels; high bicarbonate concentration).
- Liver function tests (all enzymes raised in severe starvation) and protein (decrease rare but a sign of poor prognosis).
- Electrocardiography (QT lengthening, U wave).
- Bone density (osteoporosis).

Somatization

Immediate management

Management has several strands: (1) to engage the patient in some form of dialogue; (2) to reduce further doctor visits, investigations, and so on; and (3) if possible to treat any underlying psychological disorder. It is essential that the patient feels understood: listen to the whole history of the symptoms and their impact. You are not taking a history in order to diagnose ischaemic heart disease, but so that the patient feels you have listened and understood their predicament and suffering. See the patient regularly, but not in response to symptoms. Do not say, 'Come and see me when you feel bad', but 'Come every month anyway'. In a session you will usually have to listen to some account of the symptoms and their impact, even if you can do nothing about them. It can be useful to split the session in two: spend the first 15 minutes talking about symptoms and health, and then say, 'Now let's use the time for something else', and allow the patient to set another agenda.

More specific techniques, usually following cognitive behavioural principles, have been found valuable. These usually involve some combination of cognitive work, looking at explanations for symptoms, generating alternative explanations, and looking at the links between sleep, mood, illness fears, and symptoms. This may be followed by some form of activity management programme with the intention of reducing the link between the experience of symptoms and some maladaptive behaviour pattern (such as going to bed). It is useful to be able to give sensible explanations for symptoms so that patients: (a) have an understanding of why they experience symptoms and (b) do not feel that you believe their symptoms are imaginary. Explaining the role of muscle tension in headache or chest pain, anxiety in palpitations, poor sleep and daytime fatigue, inactivity in muscle pain, hyperventilation in chest pain can all be useful.

Symptom checklists can be useful, partly to monitor progress and particularly if planning an intervention such as antidepressants, in order to check that any reported side-effects really are new. The underlying principle is to enable the patient to take responsibility for their illness and recovery (and not rely on doctors, drugs, surgical procedures, and so on), but without feeling any guilt or blame for getting ill in the first place. This is harder than it sounds.

Things not to do
If the patient has a specific illness belief ('candida', 'ME', 'chronic allergy') do not question this, even if there is no corroborating medical evidence. Never get into a confrontation, or say, 'This illness doesn't exist'. Instead, having accepted the label, move on to 'How can we help you live with the symptoms/distress' or 'How can we help you reduce your pain/disability, etc.'. Never attempt to switch the patient from a solely physical to a solely psychological model. This is both inappropriate and largely impossible. Having obtained a full history and made certain that basic investigations have been performed (such as thyroid function tests and/or ESR), do not refer to more specialists or perform more tests, unless some new indication comes along, suggestive of a different problem.

Pharmacological management
Drug therapy is not often helpful. However, contrary to conventional psychiatric teaching, there is some evidence that low-dose tricyclics can be effective for problems such as pain and sleep disorder. Many patients will be reluctant to take antidepressants, but may accept them on that basis.

Response to treatment
Most patients with somatization are seen in primary care and are usually easy to engage; they respond well to simple treatments. Cognitive behavioural treatments are successful in those with discrete disorders such as atypical chest pain, low back pain, or chronic fatigue. However, those with long illness histories, who may fulfil criteria for somatization disorder, have a poor prognosis. 'Damage limitation', long-term support, and encouragement may be indicated.

Sexual disorders
Management of sexual dysfunctions
The general management is best done with both partners (if available) and will include both sexual homework exercises and couple

relationship work. If there is no partner or the partner is unavailable, it is still possible to treat the individual, but modifications have to be made to the approach and the prognosis is more uncertain.

Behavioural approaches

The sensate focus technique of Masters and Johnson is widely used as a basic form of 'homework exercise' in most sex therapy. There is a ban on intercourse and instead a form of prolonged foreplay designed to improve communication on sexual matters and to reduce performance anxiety. The couple then progress to genital contact and to specific techniques for each specific dysfunction. For **premature ejaculation**, Semans' stop–start technique is used, stimulating the erect penis and stopping at the 'point of inevitability' just before ejaculation. For **delayed ejaculation**, the technique of penile 'super-stimulation' is recommended, perhaps with the aid of a vibrator; this is usually more successful when the man can already ejaculate in masturbation rather than when he has a total inability to ejaculate. For **erectile dysfunction**, gradual progression from sensate focus to penetration in the 'woman above' position is recommended, with a progression to physical or pharmacological approaches if necessary (see below). For **anorgasmia**, the couple is asked to practise clitoral stimulation, including the use of vibrators. For **vaginismus**, the use of finger dilatation or of graduated dilators is recommended, followed by a careful progression to intercourse. For **dyspareunia**, the treatment depends on the cause, and gynaecological procedures may be needed. In those without a physical cause sensate focus, relaxation, different positions for intercourse, and relationship therapy may be useful. For **disorders of sexual desire**, the approach is more variable, depending on the factors contributing to it: it may include couple relationship therapy, individual psychotherapy, post-traumatic counselling, anti-depressant treatment, hormone therapy, advice on lifestyle changes, and other measures.

Psychotherapeutic approaches

Psychodynamic therapy for the individual with a dysfunction is used, especially when a 'block' is reached and progress ceases. Short-term dynamic therapy may be used in the course of sex therapy, and longer-term therapy may be given in addition if other indications are present.

Cognitive therapy may be used in cases where there is depression or anxiety to be treated. In those with post-traumatic states (e.g. following rape or sexual abuse), specific post-traumatic counselling may be given.

Relationship therapy is indicated in most cases of dysfunction in couples, especially if there are resentments or tensions present. Relationship therapy is very useful in couples where one partner is more enthusiastic than the other for sex (disorders of desire).

Mechanical or pharmacological treatment

This is used mainly in **erectile dysfunction**. Penile rings and vacuum pumps can improve erections, and are acceptable to many couples.

Sildenafil (Viagra) has been introduced for the oral treatment of erectile dysfunction. It requires thorough assessment of the underlying causes, usually in a specialist setting. It is generally used for functional, rather than psychological, erectile dysfunction. It should not be prescribed in patients consuming nitrites. Yohimbine by mouth can improve the quality of erection as well as increasing sexual drive, but is not fully approved by the Committee on the Safety of Medicines. Intracavernosal injections of prostaglandin or papaverine reliably produce erections, but are less acceptable to some couples as a means of allowing intercourse. If the cavernosal blood supply is shown to be inadequate (by arteriography), surgery may be attempted to increase the arterial input.

In **premature ejaculation** it is possible to achieve some delay by utilizing a side-effect of the SSRI drugs or clomipramine. The effect is not, however, predictable and is often quite small. Vibrators are used in **female anorgasmia** and in **delayed ejaculation** in males, with variable success. Hormone replacement in postmenopausal women can reverse **atrophic vaginitis**, a frequent cause of pain and bleeding on intercourse. Hormone replacement in men is not as widely accepted and should be reserved for cases with demonstrated androgen deficiency.

Sexual deviations and gender dysphoria

If the deviation is harmful, it is usual for the police and the courts to be involved before psychiatrists. Some patients, however, come to psychiatrists first, and then ethical dilemmas can arise over disclosure. The general rule is that if there is criminal activity taking place, especially if it involves a child, the doctor is bound to break the usual rules of confidentiality and inform the social services and/or police of what has been disclosed.

Management of any deviation is much easier and treatment more likely to be successful if the patient is either self-referred or comes with a clear aim to reduce the deviant behaviour. Those who are referred by courts or who come as a result of pressure from family members or advisers are much less likely to do well.

Treatment is by behavioural, cognitive, or dynamic psychotherapy, by couple or family therapy, or by medication, in specialist centres. In cases where the patient wishes to be free of all sexual urges, the use of antilibidinal medication can be considered. Cyproterone acetate is the most satisfactory, but ethinyloestradiol and medroxyprogesterone may be used as alternatives. Ethical questions may be raised, especially in younger patients.

Management of transsexualism

It is important not to move too quickly into gender reassignment procedures, and usual to recommend that the patient should live as a member of the opposite sex for a period of 2 years, usually with the aid of hormone therapy, before any consideration of surgery.

It is then possible in selected cases to carry out gender reassignment operations with hormone therapy, but a good deal of counselling is necessary after the operation, and adjustment is variable.

Learning difficulties

Learning disability is not a disease: it does not respond to medical treatment. The appropriate treatment is that for the underlying mental condition (if any).

1. Drugs do not control primary behavioural disturbances: they may make behaviours much worse.

2. Always carry out a physical examination. Refer for medical or surgical advice if pain is apparent. General diagnostic screening should be undertaken if there are signs of physical ill-health.

3. Offer treatment appropriate to underlying mental condition (if any). Sedation may be necessary to control the violently disturbed patient; caution is necessary in view of frequent coexistence of epilepsy. Lorazepam is probably the safest sedative (2 mg orally, intravenously, or intramuscularly).

4. Do **not** initiate regular neuroleptic medication unless there are psychotic symptoms. Neuroleptic drugs should be started only by a specialist who has considered all other options.

Screening for specific syndromes of learning disability is generally pointless. Specialist investigations are best left to the specialist services. Long-term care in hospital is not an option.

Things you need to know about

Mental Health Act 1983

A working knowledge of the Mental Health Act is essential for all psychiatrists. This section summarizes some of the things you need most frequently. More details are to be found in the Code of Practice 1993[1].

Section 1 definitions

Mental disorder is defined as 'mental illness, arrested or incomplete development of mind, psychopathic disorder and any other disorder or disability of mind'.

Four categories of mental disorder are specified as follows:

1. **Mental illness:** not defined.
2. **Severe mental impairment:** 'a state of arrested or incomplete development of mind which includes severe impairment of intelligence and social functioning and is associated with abnormally aggressive or seriously irresponsible conduct on the part of the person concerned'.

---

[1] Code of Practice. Mental Health Act 1983. London: HMSO, 1993.

3. **Mental impairment:** defined in the same way as severe mental impairment except that the phrase 'severe impairment' is replaced by 'significant impairment'.

4. **Psychopathic disorder:** 'a persistent disorder or disability of mind (whether or not including significant impairment of intelligence) which results in abnormally aggressive or seriously irresponsible conduct on the part of the person concerned'.

NB: Acute intoxication, substance dependence, or sexual preference disorders alone do not qualify for these criteria.

Assessment prior to admission to hospital

As well as satisfying the criteria for mental disorder, a patient may be compulsorily admitted under the Mental Health Act in the interests of their own health, **or** safety, **or** for the protection of others.

The code of practice also says the following criteria should be considered.

- nature of illness or behaviour disorder
- patient's wishes and views
- social and family circumstances
- views of patient, relatives, and close friends about likely course of illness, the reliability of this, and any impact on them of a deterioration
- needs of family or cohabitees, and the burden on them if not admitted under the Act
- need for protection of others—including past history, risk, and reliability of others to cope
- appropriateness of guardianship
- impact of compulsory admission on patient's life after discharge
- interests of the patients's own health and whether there is any evidence that their mental health would deteriorate if no treatment were received
- reliable evidence of risk to others and its nature and degree
- willingness and ability to cope with this risk by those with whom patient lives.

If the patient is subject to the effects of sedative medication, or the short-term effects of drugs or alcohol, the **Approved Social Worker** (ASW) should wait to apply for compulsory admission until the effects have abated, unless this is not possible because of the patient's disturbed behaviour. The ASW is responsible for coordinating the process of assessment and implementing the decision for application.

The **doctor** is responsible for:

1. Deciding whether patient is suffering from mental disorder within the meaning of the Act, its seriousness, and the need for further assessment and/or treatment in hospital.

2. Specifically addressing legal criteria for admission.

3. Ensuring that a bed is available.

The doctors and ASWs should, wherever possible, consult colleagues (e.g. CPN), but retain final responsibility.

Section 2 pointers (see p. 172)

(a) Where the diagnosis and prognosis of a patient's condition is unclear.

(b) There is a need to carry out an inpatient assessment in order to formulate a treatment plan.

(c) Where a judgement is needed as to whether the patient will accept treatment on a voluntary basis following admission.

(d) Where a judgement has to be made as to whether a particular treatment proposal, which can be administered to the patient only under Part IV of the Act, is likely to be effective.

(e) Where a patient who has already been assessed, and who has previously been admitted compulsorily under the Act, is judged to have changed since the previous admission and needs further assessment.

(f) Where the patient has not previously been admitted to hospital either compulsorily or informally.

Section 3 pointers (see p. 173)

(a) Where a patient has been admitted in the past, is considered to need compulsory admission for the treatment of a mental disorder that is already known to the clinical team, and has been assessed in the recent past by that team.

(b) Where a patient already admitted under Section 2 and who is assessed as needing further medical treatment for mental disorder under the Act at the conclusion of detention under Section 2 is unwilling to remain in hospital informally and to consent to the medical treatment.

(c) Where a patient is detained under Section 2 and assessment points to a need for treatment under the Act for a period beyond the 28-day detention under Section 2. In such circumstances an application for detention under Section 3 should be made at the earliest opportunity and should not be delayed until the end of Section 2 detention. Changing a patient's detention status from Section 2 to Section 3 will not deprive them of a Mental Health Review Tribunal hearing if the change takes place after a valid application has been made to the Tribunal but before it has been heard. The patient's rights to apply for a Tribunal under Section 66(1)(b) in the first period of detention after the change of status are unaffected.

Capacity and consent to treatment

Common law applies to all patients, detained or informal. Therefore, valid consent is required from a patient before medical treatment can be given, except where the law provides authority to treat the patient without consent.

It is the personal responsibility of any doctor proposing to treat a patient to determine whether the patient has the capacity to give a valid consent. In order to have capacity an individual must be able to understand:

- the nature of the proposed treatment
- why someone has said that treatment is needed
- the treatment's principal benefits and risks
- the consequences of not receiving the proposed treatment.

A person suffering from a mental disorder is not necessarily incapable of giving consent. The legal propositions regarding this are summarized in Lord Donaldson's judgement in *Re. T. (Adult: Refusal of Medical Treatment)* (1992) All E.R. 649, 664 C.A. This presumes a capacity of an adult to refuse treatment if the reasons are 'rational or irrational, unknown or even non-existent'. An adult may be deprived of this capacity by long-term mental incapacity, retarded development, or 'temporary factors such as unconsciousness or confusion or the effects of fatigue, shock, pain or drugs'. Doctors must consider the patient's capacity, what treatment is being refused, and the circumstances in which it has arisen.

The junior may be faced with the question of capacity in two common situations:

1. A disturbed patient on a general ward who is refusing treatment.
2. A patient suffering from a mental disorder that is leading to behaviour that is an immediate serious danger to him or herself, or to other people.

In the second case, the Mental Health Act guidelines state that 'on rare occasions involving emergencies, where it is not possible immediately to apply the provisions of the MHA ... a patient ... may be given such treatment as represents the minimum necessary response to avert that danger'. In the first case, consideration should be given to the application of the Act to the patient. Both cases should ideally be discussed with seniors.

A less common situation is that of the patient with long-term incapacity who is unable to consent to treatment but does not resist it. While it is legal to treat such patients without using compulsory powers, the case of R v Bournewood Community Mental Health Trust (1998) drew attention to the problem that the rights of informal patients without capacity are not protected adequately.

Consideration should be given to detaining such patients so that a Tribunal can review treatment decisions.

Consent to treatment (Part IV of the Mental Health Act)

This applies to:

- treatments for mental disorder
- all formal patients except those who are detained under Sections 4, 5, 35, 135, and 136, subject to guardianship or conditionally discharged: these patients have the right to refuse treatment as have informal patients, except in emergencies

Part IV states that:

(i) any treatment can be given without the patient's consent unless the Mental Health Act or DHSS regulations specify otherwise

(ii) under Section 57, psychosurgery and treatments specified in DHSS regulations as giving rise to special concern can be given only if:

   (a) the patient consents; and

   (b) a multidisciplinary panel appointed by the Mental Health Act Commission confirms that the patient's consent is valid; and

   (c) the doctor on the multidisciplinary panel certifies that the treatment should be given; before doing so the doctor must consult two people, one a nurse and the other neither a nurse nor a doctor, who have been concerned with the patient's treatment.

   Note: As the treatments specified in section 57 give rise to particular concern, this section applies to all formal and informal patients.

(iii) under Section 58, certain treatments can be given only if:

   (a) the patient consents; or

   (b) an independent doctor appointed by the Mental Health Act Commission confirms that treatment should be given; before doing so the doctor must consult two people, one a nurse and the other neither a nurse nor a doctor, who have been concerned with the patient's treatment.

Section 58 applies to treatments named in DHSS regulations (including ECT). Medication can be given without the patient's consent for 3 months; after that it is subject to the safeguards laid down in Section 58.

Note: Under Section 62, any treatment for mental disorder can be given without consent in specific emergencies, subject to restrictions when a treatment is irreversible or hazardous.

Table 11.1 Sections of the Mental Health Act

SECTION	DURATION	APPLICATION	PROCEDURES	DISCHARGE
2 Admission for assessment	28 days maximum	ASW or nearest relative. Applicant must have seen patient within the previous 14 days	Two doctors must confirm that: (a) patient is suffering from mental disorder of a nature or degree that warrants detention in hospital for assessment (or assessment followed by medical treatment) for at least a limited period; and (b) the patient ought to be detained in the interests of his or her own health or safety or with a view to the protection of others	By any of the following: (a) RMO (b) hospital managers (c) nearest relative who must give 72 hours' notice. RMO can prevent nearest relative from discharging patient by making a report to the hospital managers d) MHRT. Patient can apply to a tribunal within the first 14 days of detention*
4 Admission for assessment in cases of emergency	72 hours maximum	ASW or nearest relative. Applicant must have seen patient within the previous 24 hours	One doctor must confirm that: (a) it is of 'urgent necessity' for the patient to be admitted and detained under Section 2; and (b) waiting for a second doctor to confirm the need for an admission under Section 2 would cause 'undesirable delay'	

| 3 | Admission for treatment | 6 months, renewable for a further 6 months, then for 1 year at a time | By ASW or nearest relative or in cases where it is not 'reasonably practicable' to consult nearest relative consent is displaced by County Court | Two doctors must confirm that: (a) patient is suffering from one of the four specified categories of mental disorder, a nature or degree that makes it appropriate for him or her to receive medical treatment in hospital; and (b) if patient is suffering from psychopathic disorder or mental impairment, such treatment is likely to 'alleviate or prevent a deterioration' of his or her condition; and (c) it is necessary for the patient's own health or safety or for the protection of others that he or she receives such treatment and it cannot be provided unless the patient is detained under this section | By any of the following: (a) RMO (b) hospital managers (c) nearest relative who must give 72 hours' notice. RMO can prevent nearest relative from discharging patient by making a report to the hospital managers d) MHRT. Patient can apply to a tribunal within 6 months of admission and during each subsequent renewal period |

Renewal: Under Section 20, RMO can renew a Section 3 detention order if original criteria still apply and treatment is likely to 'alleviate or prevent a deterioration' of patient's condition. In cases where patient is suffering from mental illness or severe mental impairment but treatment is not likely to alleviate or prevent a deterioration of his or her condition, detention may still be renewed if the patient is unlikely to be able to care for him or herself, to obtain the care needed, or to guard him or herself again serious exploitation.

Table 11.1 (Continued)

SECTION	DURATION	APPLICATION	PROCEDURES	DISCHARGE
5 (2)	72 hours maximum	Doctor of informal inpatient's treatment or nominated deputy (usually on-call doctor)	Reports to hospital managers that application for compulsory admission 'ought to be made'. Applies to inpatients being treated for physical disorders but not those seen in accident and emergency. The nominated deputy should contact the nominated doctor or another consultant before using Section 5 (2) where possible	Should be converted to Section 2 or 3, or rescinded as soon as possible

136 If it appears to a police officer that a person in a public place is 'suffering from mental disorder' and is 'in immediate need of care or control', the officer can take that person to a 'place of safety', usually a hospital. Section 136 lasts for a maximum of 72 hours so that person can be examined by a doctor and interviewed by the ASW, and 'any necessary arrangements' made for treatment or care.

135 If there is reasonable cause to suspect that a person is suffering from mental disorder and:

(a) is being ill-treated or neglected or not kept under proper control; or

(b) is unable to care for him or herself and lives alone, magistrates issues a warrant authorizing a police officer (with a doctor and ASW) to enter any premises where the person is believed to be and remove him or her to a place of safety.

Patients involved in criminal proceedings (Part III)

Hospital order (Section 37)

Duration   Initially this lasts for 6 months, renewable for a further 6 months, then yearly.

Procedure   Can be made by a Crown or Magistrates' Court in the case of a convicted offender in place of a prison sentence. (Offences include manslaughter but not murder). Magistrates' court need not record a conviction if satisfied that the offender was suffering from mental illness or severe mental impairment at the time of the offence.

A hospital order requires evidence from two doctors that:

• the offender is suffering from one of the specified categories of mental disorder of a nature and degree that makes detention for medical treatment appropriate; and

• if suffering from psychopathic disorder or mental impairment, such treatment is likely to 'alleviate or prevent a deterioration of the person's condition; and

• taking into account all the relevant circumstances, a hospital order is most appropriate.

Discharge   By RMO, hospital manager, or MHRT (one application allowed between 6 and 12 months, and then yearly; the case is automatically reconsidered by the MHRT 3 years after the last tribunal referral).

Restriction order (Section 41)

Duration   May be specified by court or without limit.

Procedure   Crown Court only after imposition of a hospital order if:

• this is necessary to protect the public from 'serious harm'; and

• at least one of the doctors who made recommendations for the hospital order gave evidence orally.

Discharge   By either Home Secretary or MHRT (rules as for Section 37). Most Section 37/41 patients who are discharged by the Home Office or MHRT are 'conditionally discharged', meaning Section 41 remains in place. If conditions set by the Home Office are broken, the Home Office may recall the person to hospital, where they revert to Section 37 or 41.

Police and Criminal Evidence Act 1984

The Police and Criminal Evidence Act 1984 was designed to regulate police conduct and the admissibility of evidence in court. Sections 53–65 deal with the treatment and questioning of people in police custody.

If a detained person appears mentally disordered (defined according to Mental Health Act 1983 criteria), police must ask an 'appropriate adult' to come to the police station. The concern is that a mentally disordered person will give evidence that is unreliable and/or self-incriminatory. Similar provision is made for juveniles. This does not apply in emergencies (e.g. where the risk to others can be reduced by questioning someone immediately).

The 'appropriate adult' may be a relative or carer, or someone who has worked with mentally disordered people, but it cannot be the person's solicitor. The adult cannot be employed by the police. The Code of Practice states that a well-informed professional may be preferable to an ill-informed relative, but also that the person's choice of adult is to be respected.

The 'appropriate adult' should be present during searches and questioning, observe fairness of interviews, advise the person being questioned, and facilitate communication. The person being questioned is entitled to consult privately with the appropriate adult at any time (this is often not respected).

The Act also makes provision that mentally disordered detainees should not be subject to voluntary searches (because of doubts about the quality of their consent). In all cases, the more stringent procedures that cover involuntary searches must be applied. If confessions made by mentally disordered people are used in evidence against them in court, the judge must refer to the unreliability of such confessions in his or her summing up.

Children's Act 1989

Emergency Protection Order (for children)

Sometimes a psychiatric assessment of a child will reveal a dangerous and harmful situation so that emergency care is needed. If so, the duty social worker should be contacted urgently, as well as the consultant in charge of the case.

The Emergency Protection Order replaced the old Place of Safety Order under the Children and Young Persons Act 1969. It was felt, following the Cleveland Inquiry, that the place of safety order was used rather too indiscriminately, and that parental rights were too easily infringed.

An application for an Emergency Protection Order can be made under Section 44 of the Children Act 1989. The court will make an order if there are reasonable grounds to believe that the child is likely to suffer significant harm, or cannot be seen in circumstances where he or she might be suffering significant harm. The court will wish to know why a child should be removed as a matter of urgency, and why parental cooperation should be dispensed with at this stage.

The duration is limited to 8 days, with possible extension for a further 7 days. Applications to lift the order can be made between 72 hours and 8 days.

The person obtaining the order has limited parental responsibility. The court will decide about parental contact, and medical and psychiatric assessment.

The new Mental Health Act

In December 2000, a White Paper outlined the modifications now proposed for reform of the Mental Health Act 1983. There are no longer to be four categories of mental disorder; the definition is '*any disability or disorder of mind or brain, whether temporary or permanent, which results in an impairment or disturbance of mental functioning*'. The intention is to move away from the criterion of 'treatability', which limited use of the previous Act. Someone with a personality disorder who poses a serious risk of significant harm to others may be detained under the new provisions. There are three stages in the framework of legislation.

Stage 1: Initial use of compulsory powers

If compulsory powers are to be used to detain the patient, the recommendation must be made by two doctors and a social worker or other mental health professional who has received specific training in use of the legislation.

- The mental disorder must be 'sufficiently serious to warrant further assessment and urgent treatment'; and
- 'without intervention the patient is likely to be at risk of serious harm—including deterioration of health—or pose a significant risk to others';
- the patient must be resisting—or considered likely to resist—proposals for assessment or treatment, or not complying with an existing treatment programme.

The formal procedure can be triggered by a request to a Trust from the patient, from his or her carer or GP, or from a criminal justice agency. The Trust may arrange for such preliminary examination to be made by an appropriate specialist service. One of the doctors making the recommendation will work in the service providing care and be approved under the new legislation, while the other may be the patient's GP, be from another specialist mental health service, or be 'another doctor approved under the new legislation'. The third person will be a social worker or another approved mental health professional who has expertise in mental disorder and who is responsible for coordinating the examination process. They will consider alternatives to compulsory treatment that may be locally available, and will also coordinate the next steps if compulsory treatment is to continue beyond 3 days.

Stage 2: Formal assessment and initial treatment

A full assessment must be made to determine the patient's health and social care needs within 3 days of admission and, if the patient is to remain in hospital a **written care plan** must be prepared. If the first two of the above conditions are no longer met, the patient may no longer be treated using the compulsory powers.

Initial use of compulsory powers can be extended to a period of 28 days, after which time continuous use of such powers can be made only by a Mental Health Tribunal.

Stage 3: Care and treatment orders

The Tribunal may make a first care and assessment order for 6 months; and subsequent orders for up to 12 months. The order will authorize treatments specified in the care plan. The patient may request the Tribunal to review his or her need for continuing care using compulsory powers once during the initial period, and once in any succeeding period of 12 months. To continue to detain a patient who has been detained in his or her best interest, the care plan must be of direct benefit to the patient, and in those where the risk is primarily to others the plan must treat the underlying mental disorder or manage the behaviours arising from the disorder.

The care programme approach

The care programme approach (CPA) was introduced in 1991 to provide a framework for effective mental health care. It aims to guide good clinical practice and to prevent patients from 'slipping through the net'. The key principles are applicable to all service users, even those who require an intervention only by a single discipline.

Its four main elements are:

1. *Assessment of health and social care needs*: The systematic assessment begins with a good psychiatric history. Most patients with severe mental illness will have a wide range of needs, and a full assessment will involve information obtained from informants: family, friends, professional and non-professional carers. It is now mandatory that assessment of mental health needs be integrated with that of social needs in a single care coordination approach. A joint assessment process prevents duplication for the user and carer, and ensures that the services allocated from whichever source match need.

2. *A written care plan*: For patients requiring multidisciplinary input, a care plan should be agreed at a ward round or CPA meeting with everyone who will be involved in implementing it. The plan should be agreed as far as possible with the patient, and with carers. For other patients, this might simply involve a plan for outpatient treatment being written in the notes following assessment, although even this should be discussed and agreed with the patient.

3. *Care coordinator*: The care coordinator has responsibility for the coordination of the care programme. He or she is responsible for keeping in close contact with the patient, and for advising the other members of the care team of changes in the circumstances of the

patient that might require review or modification of the care plan. The care coordinator should be the professional with the closest relationship with the patient; this will often be a CPN or social worker, but could be the psychiatrist in training.

4. *Ongoing reviews*: Review and evaluation of care planning should be regarded as an ongoing process. There is no required set period for review, but at each review meeting the date of the next review must be set and recorded. However, any member of the care team or the patient or carer must be able to ask for a review at any time. If the team decides that a review is not necessary, the reasons for this must be recorded. Trusts should ensure that a system is in place to collect data on all service users whose care is managed through the CPA.

Who should receive the CPA?

To establish consistency of practice, from April 2001 services have been required to deliver the CPA according to two levels: standard or enhanced. The characteristics of people receiving either form are listed below.

Standard CPA

- Require the support or intervention of one agency or discipline or low-key support from more than one agency or discipline.
- They are more able to manage their mental health problems.
- They have an informal support network.
- They pose little danger to themselves or others.
- They are more likely to maintain appropriate contact with services .

Enhanced CPA

- They have multiple care needs, including housing, employment, etc., requiring inter-agency coordination.
- They are willing to cooperate with only one professional or agency, but they have multiple care needs.
- They may be in contact with a number of agencies.
- They are likely to require more frequent and intensive interventions.
- They are more likely to have mental health problems coexisting with other problems, such as substance misuse.
- They are more likely to be at risk of harming themselves or others.
- They are more likely to disengage with services.

Supervised discharge

Supervised discharge was introduced by the Mental Health (Patients in the Community) Act 1995, which amended the Mental Health Act 1983.

Criteria for the application

The application is made by the RMO to the provider unit managers. The patient will have already satisfied the conditions for detention under the sections given above, and in addition the RMO believes that there will be a substantial risk of serious harm to the patient or to the safety of other people if the patient does not receive aftercare on discharge from hospital, and that the powers of supervised discharge are likely to help ensure that the patient receives aftercare. The aftercare will be delivered according to enhanced CPA.

The application by the RMO must be supported by applications from another doctor approved under Section 12(2), who could be the consultant providing community care (the 'Community RMO') if different from the RMO, or the GP, and from an approved social worker. The application must include an agreed care plan.

The supervised discharge takes effect only once the patient is discharged from both hospital and detention, so it does not apply while the patient is on leave of absence (Section 17). The patient has a right of appeal to a Mental Health Review Tribunal (but not to a managers' hearing). Supervised discharge lasts for 6 months, and the RMO can apply to renew it for a further 6 months, then for a year at a time.

Responsibilities of the services

The RMO must consult the patient, the hospital team, the proposed supervisor (community key worker), informal carers, the nearest relative, and social services about the application for supervised discharge. The care plan must be agreed with local social services, and should be agreed with others who will be involved in implementing it. The patient must be informed; he or she does not have to agree to be supervised, but in practice the care plan may be impossible to implement if the patient does not cooperate at all. The supervisor must monitor the provision of the care plan, and the RMO must provide psychiatric treatment and, if the care plan is not working, must consult the relevant parties to revise the plan.

Requirements of the patient

The patient can be required to reside in a particular place, to attend at set times for medical treatment, occupation, education, or training, and the supervisor must be allowed access to the place of residence to see the patient.

Powers of the supervisor

The supervisor has the 'power to take and convey' the patient, to home or to a place of treatment, with police or ambulance support if necessary. This can be done only if it is likely to result in the patient then cooperating with treatment, as the supervisor cannot prevent the patient from leaving the place of treatment as soon as he or she arrives, and the patient cannot be forced to accept treatment. If necessary, the patient could be assessed for detention in hospital under Section 3.

Benefits

There may be a small group of patients who are currently very difficult to care for who will respond to the more assertive treatment the supervisor can provide using supervised discharge.

Limitations

Although the procedure is elaborate, the powers are limited and may be ineffective, if the patient is determined not to cooperate with the care plan. They may restrict civil liberties without making it possible to deliver better care.

Needs assessment

The assessment of need by both social and health services is a requirement of the care programme approach. Social services are also required under the NHS and Community Care Act 1990 to provide an assessment of social care needs to all those who require one, including those with mental disorder, and these types of assessment should overlap as much as is practicable.

Defining needs

Needs can be defined on a population or individual basis, and from the perspectives of politicians, clinicians, carers, and patients—clearly, these will differ. A working definition of need in the sense in which it is used in the CPA is that a need exists where the patient 'is able in some way to benefit from care', where this care is medical or social. The needs are not limited to the care that happens to be available; a broader definition of need may suggest services that could be developed.

Need in severe mental illness

The needs for care of the severely mentally ill are often considerable, and involve physical, mental, and social needs. While a good psychiatric history and examination should identify many of these, some, particularly social care needs, may be insufficiently covered. A standardized instrument, the Camberwell Assessment of Needs (CAN)[2] identifies 22 areas of need to be explored in a full assessment (see Table 11.2). The instrument enables problems in these areas to be

---

[2] Copies of the Camberwell Assessment of Need are obtainable from Health Services Research Department, Institute of Psychiatry, De Crespigny Park, Denmark Hill, London SE5 8AF, UK. Tel: 020 7919 2610. Fax: 020 7277 1462.

Table 11.2 Areas of need in patients with severe mental illness

Accommodation	Alcohol
Food	Drugs
Household skills	Company of others
Self-care	Intimate relationships
Occupation	Sexual expression
Physical health	Child care
Psychotic symptoms	Basic education
Information about condition and treatment	Telephone
Psychological distress	Transport
Safety to self	Money
Safety to others	Welfare benefits

rated from interviews with the patient, or by the key worker, in about half an hour, and distinguishes unmet needs from those already met by help from informal carers or statutory services.

Community visits

This section discusses some practical aspects of patient contact by psychiatrists in non-medical settings. Community visiting is highly informative, enjoyable, and appreciated by patients and carers. Visiting people at home provides an invaluable insight into the social context of the patient's psychopathology and their level of functioning. The techniques of assessment and management described in this book are equally applicable outside the hospital, for example in the patient's home, a hostel or day centre, a police station, or even the street. However, these settings are less predictable than the clinic or ward and more emotionally demanding. As a consequence some special considerations apply.

Patients may be seen in the community as part of the assessment process, for planned treatment or review, as an emergency intervention in a crisis, or in a formal Mental Health Act assessment. Family assessment and intervention may usefully be carried out in the home. Care programme approach reviews are often held in non-medical settings. With the possible exception of the traditional consultant domiciliary consultation requested by the GP, all home visiting should be part of the work of the multidisciplinary community mental health team. Home assessments by psychiatrists should generally be carried out with colleagues in the team. Home treatment and review will be part of a previously agreed care plan. Emergency assessments should be carried out in accordance with locally agreed operational policies or protocols. 'Good practice' in the conduct of a Mental Health Act assessment is set out in a Code of Practice 1993[3], with which, for

---

[3] Code of Practice. Mental Health Act 1983. London: HMSO, 1993.

medicolegal reasons, all psychiatrists in England and Wales should be familiar.

Planning the visit

The reasons for and expected outcome of any community visit should be identified. If hospital admission is the expected outcome of an emergency assessment, the availability of a bed should be confirmed before setting out. Alternatively, the possibilities of intensive community support to an acutely ill patient should be explored before the visit. If the patient is likely to require medication, is a prescription available? A mobile telephone may be helpful if complex arrangements will have to be made. The visiting psychiatrist should have the maximum possible information. Before carrying out an emergency or new patient assessment, informants should be contacted by phone. Any documentation should be sought and read. It is helpful to know the exact nature of the community concerns are before any doorstep assessment:

- What is the alleged psychopathology?
- What abnormal behaviours have others reported?
- What are the patient's documented risks to self or others?

The patient should generally be given notice of the visit, which should preferably take place at a mutually agreed time. The reason for and conduct of any unannounced visit should be very clearly thought out in advance. The journey to a visit should be planned: find out exactly where to go, how long it will take, and where to park. At night, take a torch. If a colleague, carer, or the police are to attend the visit, a rendezvous should be agreed. Arrangements for access to the home should be identified before the visit: if access is impossible, consideration should be given to the use of Section 135 of the Mental Health Act. This requires the involvement of an Approved Social Worker colleague.

Safety

The possible risks of any community visit should always be considered:

- Is the patient (and family) known to services?
- Is there any past history of violence or aggression?

If there are any concerns about safety, the psychiatrist should visit with a colleague from the team, the GP, or a person previously known to the patient. Unobtrusive police presence may be advisable during a Mental Health Act assessment. As a general principle, **another team member should know about any community visit**—community staff have been held hostage! If, during a visit, staff feel unsafe, they should not hesitate to retreat. If, following a strategic retreat, there are concerns about the safety of other household members, some plan of action should be drawn up, for example a follow-up telephone call or contact with the police.

Carrying out a visit

Any home visit should be carried out in a calm and confident manner. The psychiatrist is often expected to take the lead in the conduct of the visit, and should therefore be clear what the task of the visit is. Communications should be clear and unambiguous. Certain courtesies should be observed, for example seeking permission to enter the house and establishing with the patient and any carer the purpose of the interview, its likely duration, and where it should be carried out. Introductions should be made. The composition of the household should be established; visitors should be sensitive to the needs of children in the home. When carers are present, they should be allowed to contribute to the discussion of the patient's problems, although rights to confidentiality should always be considered. It may be appropriate to interview the patient and carers separately. It is quite reasonable to ask the patient to turn off their television or remove their pet from the interview setting. If one aim of the visit is to assess the patient's level of functioning and home environment, this should be carried out sensitively, although it is usually appropriate to share any concerns about their welfare with the patient. At the end of the visit a plan of further care should be negotiated with the patient and carer. Preferably, the timing of any further home visit or outpatient contact should be agreed. Details of a contact person, address, and telephone number should be offered to the patient and carer. The referrer should be formally contacted following an assessment, which should be recorded in the case notes. It will often be helpful to carry out a short debriefing session with any accompanying colleague immediately after the visit, both to clarify the outcome of the visit and for emotional support.

Emergency and Mental Health Act assessments

The conduct of emergency assessments will reflect the treatment paradigms, resource base, and policies of the local service. There may be a Crisis Intervention Team capable of responding to requests from GPs, patients and carers, and community agencies for the assessment and treatment of people in psychosocial crisis. A service may be able to provide 24-hour home care for acutely psychotic patients as an alternative to inpatient admission, or may only be able to offer institution of treatment, intermittent home visits, and outpatient attendance. The general principles are set out above: careful planning (the more important, the more acute the situation), consideration of personal safety, calm conduct throughout the intervention, and appropriate follow-up. Access arrangements are crucial to effective emergency interventions.

Assessments for admission under the Mental Health Act should generally follow the 'good practice' guidelines set out in the Code of

Practice, or its equivalent in other jurisdictions. The Code of Practice not only amplifies the criteria for compulsory admission set out in the Mental Health Act, but provides detail about the appropriate conduct of the assessment. Mental Health Act assessments are often unnecessarily chaotic and distressing for patient, carers, and staff involved. Although a rapid response to a perceived crisis is often demanded, careful planning is always appropriate. The ASW has 'overall responsibility for coordinating the process of assessment and, where he decides to make an application, for implementing the decision' (Code of Practice 2.10). The psychiatrist (always approved under Section 12 of the Mental Health Act) may wish to review these plans before the assessment and should usually have made arrangements for the patient's admission to an appropriately staffed ward in the anticipation of a decision to admit either under the Mental Health Act or informally. An ambulance and, if necessary, the police should be in attendance. Assessment should be carried out jointly by the recommending doctors (the psychiatrist and usually the GP) and the ASW 'unless good reasons prevent it' (Code of Practice 2.2). The role of the ASW is spelt out in detail (2.11–2.17). The medical examination requires 'direct personal examination of the patient's mental state' and 'consideration of all available relevant medical information' (2.20). Examining doctors 'should always discuss the patient with each other' (2.21).

Although the majority of compulsory admissions 'require prompt action to be taken', the ASW has up to 14 days from first seeing the patient to make an application (2.26). Any decision not to make an application should be accompanied by plans to implement appropriate alternative arrangements. The ASW also has a duty to inform the nearest relative of the reasons for not making an application and their right to apply (2.27).

Home visits with elderly patients

If the patient is being assessed at home, some inspection of the home circumstances should be made. This is an important part of evaluating the degree of risk posed to the patient (and possibly others). Remember that self-neglect is not diagnostic of any particular disorder and can occur in severe functional illness as well as dementia.

- Is the dwelling in a good state of repair and decoration?
- Is it secure?
- Are gas, electricity, and water connected?
- Is there adequate heating and lighting?
- Is the gas ever left on unlit?
- If the patient smokes, is there evidence of the careless use of lighted cigarettes?

- Is the patient able to call for help if necessary (e.g. via a centralized alarm system)?
- Is there enough food in the home to make, at least, small snacks/hot drinks?
- Is there evidence of urinary or faecal incontinence?
- Are any pets well cared for?

Appendix 1
The AUDIT questionnaire

Circle the number that comes closest to the patient's answer.

1. **How often do you have a drink containing alcohol?**
   (0) Never   (1) Monthly or less
   (2) 2–4 times a month   (3) 2–3 times a week
   (4) 4 or more times a week

2.[a] **How many drinks containing alcohol do you have on a typical day when you are drinking? (Code number of standard drinks)**
   (0) 1 or 2   (1) 3 or 4   (2) 5 or 6
   (3) 7 or 8   (4) 10 or more

3. **How often do you have six or more drinks on one occasion?**
   (0) Never   (1) Less than monthly   (2) Monthly
   (3) Weekly   (4) Daily or almost daily

4. **How often during the past year have you found that you were not able to stop drinking once you had started?**
   (0) Never   (1) Less than monthly   (2) Monthly
   (3) Weekly   (4) Daily or almost daily

5. **How often during the past year have you failed to do what was normally expected from you because of drinking?**
   (0) Never   (1) Less than monthly   (2) Monthly
   (3) Weekly   (4) Daily or almost daily

6. **How often during the past year have you needed a first drink in the morning to get yourself going after a heavy drinking session?**
   (0) Never   (1) Less than monthly   (2) Monthly
   (3) Weekly   (4) Daily or almost daily

7. **How often during the past year have you had a feeling of guilt or remorse after drinking?**

(0) Never   (1) Less than monthly   (2) Monthly
(3) Weekly   (4) Daily or almost daily

8. **How often during the past year have you been unable to remember what happened the night before because you had been drinking?**

(0) Never   (1) Less than monthly   (2) Monthly
(3) Weekly   (4) Daily or almost daily

9. **Have you or someone else been injured as a result of your drinking?**

(0) No   (1) Yes, but not in the last year
(4) Yes, during the last year

10. **Has a relative or friend or a doctor or other health worker been concerned about your drinking or suggested you cut down?**

(0) No   (1) Yes, but not in the last year
(4) Yes, during the last year

---

[a]In determining the response categories, it has been assumed that one 'drink' contains 10 g alcohol. In countries where the alcohol content of a standard drink differs by more than 25% from 10 g, the response category should be modified accordingly.

Appendix 2
Mini-Mental State Examination

			Score	points
Orientation				
1. What is the	Year?		.....	1
	Season?		.....	1
	Date?		.....	1
	Day?		.....	1
	Month ?		.....	1
2. Where are we?	Country?		.....	1
	County?		.....	1
	Town?		.....	1
	Hospital?		.....	1
	Floor?		.....	1

Registration

3. Name three objects, one per second (e.g. BALL, FLAG, TREE).
   Then ask the patient all three after you have said them.
   Give one point for each correct answer.
   Repeat the words until patient learns all three   3

Attention and concentration

4. Spell 'world' backwards: D L R O W   5

Recall

5. Ask for the names of the three objects learned in Q3.
   Give one point for each correct answer.   3

Language

6. Point to a pencil and a watch.
   Ask the patient to name them as you point.   2

7. Ask the patient to repeat 'No ifs, ands, or buts' 1

8. Ask the patient to read and obey the following:
CLOSE YOUR EYES 1

9. Ask the patient to carry out a three-stage command:
'Take the paper in your right hand, fold it in half, and
put it on the floor.' 3

10. Ask the patient to write a sentence of their own.
(The sentence should contain a subject and an object
and should make sense. Ignore spelling errors in scoring.) 1

11. Ask the patient to copy a design (two overlapping
pentagons).
Give one point if all sides and angles are preserved
and the intersecting sides form a quadrangle. 1

Total **30**

After Folstein et al (1975) *J Psychiatr Res* 12:189.

Abbreviated Mental Test Scoring

Hodkinson M (1972)
Evaluation of a mental test score for assessment of mental impairment
in the elderly
Age and Ageing **1** 233–238

1. age (must be correct to score)

2. time (to nearest hour)

3. Now give them an address for recall, (3 items only—e.g. 98,
Primrose Hill, Wimbledon—*repeated by the patient to ensure that
it has been heard correctly*—don't score yet

4. year (must be correct)

5. where are we?

6. Recognition of two people (usually the doctor and the carer)

7. Date of birth (they must give date, month and year to score)

8. Year of world war (must be correct year of starting and stopping)

9. Name of present monarch

10. Count backwards from 20 to 1 (each number from 20 back to 1
has to be in order—one missed number; no score)

Now ask them to recall the address given as "3" (2+ items recalled
scores the point).

Scoring is one mark for each exactly correct (Scoring is generally
accepted as 6 or below as indicating probable dementia. However a
score of 7 or 8 should be treated with caution and repeated).

Appendix 3
The 'SAD PERSONS' scale and the Risk–Rescue Rating Scale

Table A3.1 The 'SAD PERSONS' scale

S Sex is male
A Age is older than 45 or younger than 19 years
D Depression
P Previous attempts
E Ethanol abuse
R Rational thinking loss (particularly psychosis)
S Social support is lacking
O Organized plan
N No spouse
S Sickness (physical illness, especially if painful)

Each positive item receives a score of 1. A flexible use of the following evaluation can be helpful:
- *Score 0–2*: Low risk. Discharge and outpatient follow-up.
- *Score 3–4*: Moderate risk. Close monitoring as outpatient. Consider admission.
- *Score 5–6*: High risk. Admission is advised, especially if support from environment seems uncertain.
- *Score 7–10*: Very high risk of suicide. Admission required.

From Patterson et al (1983).

Table A3.2 The Risk–Rescue Rating Scale

Risk factors	Rescue factors
Agent used	*Location*
1. Ingestion, cutting, stabbing	3. Familiar
2. Drowning, asphyxiation, strangulation	2. Non-familiar, non-remote
3. Jumping, shooting	1. Remote
Impaired consciousness	*Person initiating rescue[a]*
1. None in evidence	3. Key person
2. Confusion, semi-coma	2. Professional
3. Coma, deep coma	1. Passer-by
Lesions/toxicity	*Probability of discovery by any rescuer*
1. Mild	3. High, almost certain
2. Moderate	2. Uncertain discovery
3. Severe	1. Accidental discovery
Reversibility	*Accessibility to rescue*
1. Good, complete recovery expected	3. Asks for help
2. Fair, recovery expected with time	2. Drops clues
3. Poor, residuals expected if recovery	1. Does not ask for help
Treatment required	*Delay until discovery[b]*
1. First aid, E. W. care	3. Immediate, 1 hour
2. Hospital admission, routine treatment	2. Less than 4 hours
3. Intensive care, special treatment	1. More than 4 hours
Total risk points =	**Total rescue points =**
Risk score	**Rescue score**
5 = High risk (13–15 risk points)	1 = Least rescuable (5–7 rescue points)
4 = High moderate (11–12 risk points)	2 = Low moderate (8–9 rescue points)
3 = Moderate (9–10 risk points)	3 = Moderate (10–11 rescue points)
2 = Low moderate (7–8 risk points)	4 = High moderate (12–13 rescue points)
1 = Low risk (5–6 risk points)	5 = Most rescuable (14–15 rescue points)

[a]Self-rescue automatically yields a rescue score of 5

[b]If there is undue delay in obtaining treatment after discovery, reduce the final rescue score by one point

This scale helps to assess the 'lethality' of a given parasuicide/DSH case. It does so by estimating the ratio between risk of the behaviour and likelihood of rescue.

Risk–Rescue Score = $A \times 100/A + B$, where A = risk score and B = rescue score. Thus the minimum risk–rescue score is 17 for a 'low lethality' self-harm behaviour. The maximum risk–rescue score is 83 for a 'high lethality' self-harm case.

From Weissman and Worden (1972).

Appendix 4
Antipsychotic drugs

Table A4.1 Antipsychotic drugs

Drug	Chemical group	Dose range (daily dose) Single daily dose unless stated (*)	Alternative licensed indications	Adverse effects (See data sheet for full details/ Appendix 6 for comparison)	Interactions	Cost
Chlorpromazine	Phenothiazine (Gp I—aliphatic)	25–1000 mg	Anxiety, nausea, agitation, hiccup, induction of hypothermia, violence, autism	Extrapyramidal effects, anticholinergic, sedation, hypotension, hypothermia, endocrine disorders, convulsions, jaundice, ECG change, blood dyscrasias	Sedatives, lithium, anticholinergics, antiepileptics, sulphonylureas, cimetidine, antidepressants, dopamine (ant)agonists	+

(Continued)

Table A4.1 (Continued)

Drug	Chemical group	Dose range (daily dose) Single daily dose unless stated (*)	Alternative licensed indications	Adverse effects (See data sheet for full details/ Appendix 6 for comparison)	Interactions	Cost
Promazine	Phenothiazine (Gp I—aliphatic)	400–800 mg	Agitation and restlessness in elderly NB: Weak antipsychotic	As chlorpromazine	As chlorpromazine	+
Thioridazine	Phenothiazine (Gp II-piperidine)	150–800 mg	Because of the risk of increased QTc, thioridazine should only be used as a second-line treatment for adult patients with schizophrenia. The use in children or elderly is contraindicated	As chlorpromazine + pigmented retinopathy, ejaculatory dysfunction	As chlorpromazine	+
Fluphenazine	Phenothiazine (Gp III—piperazine)	1–20 mg	Agitation, anxiety, violence	As chlorpromazine + depression reported	As chlorpromazine	+
Perphenazine	Phenothiazine (Gp III—piperazine)	12–24 mg	Agitation, severe anxiety, violence	As chlorpromazine	As chlorpromazine	+

Trifluoperazine	Phenothiazine (Gp III—piperazine)	10–50 mg (est.) (maximum dose not stated by manufacturers)	Agitation, severe anxiety, violence	As chlorpromazine	As chlorpromazine	+
Flupenthixol	Thioxanthine	6–18 mg	Depressive illness (low dose)	As chlorpromazine	As chlorpromazine	+
Zuclopenthixol	Thioxanthine	20–150 mg	None	As chlorpromazine	As chlorpromazine	+
Haloperidol	Butyrophenone	1.5–30 mg	Agitation, severe anxiety, violence, tics, nausea, hiccup, mania, Gilles de la Tourette disease	As chlorpromazine	As chlorpromazine + fluoxetine, astemizole, terfenadine	+
Droperidol	Butyrophenone	20–120 mg (*qds)	The manufacturer has withdrawn this product from the UK market because of the risk of increased QTc	As chlorpromazine + depression	As chlorpromazine	++
Benperidol	Butyrophenone	0.25–1.5 mg(*bd)	Deviant social/sexual behaviour NB: Not licensed for schizophrenia/psychoses	As chlorpromazine	As chlorpromazine	++

(Continued)

Table A4.1 (Continued)

Drug	Chemical group	Dose range (daily dose) Single daily dose unless stated (*)	Alternative licensed indications	Adverse effects (See data sheet for full details/ Appendix 6 for comparison)	Interactions	Cost
Sulpiride	Substituted benzamide	400–2400 mg (*bd)	None	As chlorpromazine; jaundice and skin reactions less common, less sedation, hypotension	As chlorpromazine	++
Pimozide	Diphenylbutylpiperidine	2–20 mg	Mania, hypocondriacal psychosis	As chlorpromazine + serious cardiac arrhythmias (monitor plasma potassium), depression	As chlorpromazine + diuretics, any cardioactive drug—this include other antipsychotics and tricyclics	+
Loxapine	Dibenzoxazepine	20–250 mg (*bd)	None	As chlorpromazine + nausea, dyspnoea, ptosis, polydipsia, paraesthesia. Few endocrine effects reported	As chlorpromazine	++

Risperidone	Benzisoxazole	2–16 mg	None	As chlorpromazine + agitation, abdominal pain, fatigue, anxiety, nausea, rhinitis	As chlorpromazine	+++
Sertindole	Imidazolidinone	12–24 mg/day	None	As chlorpromazine + nasal congestion, reduced ejaculatory volume	As chlorpromazine + all drugs which inhibit CYP2D6, e.g. fluoxetine, paroxetine	+++
Clozapine	Dibenzodiazepine	25–900 mg (*bd)	None	As chlorpromazine + hypersalivation, delerium, incontinence, myocarditis, neutropenia, fatal agranulocytosis (see Appendix 7)	As chlorpromazine + all drugs that depress leucopoiesis, e.g. cytotoxic agents, sulphonamides, chloramphenicol, carbamazepine, phenothiazines. Fluoxetine and risperidone increase clozapine plasma levels	++++
Olanzapine	Thienobenzodiazepine	5–20 mg	None	Sedation, weight gain, hypotension, anticholinergic effects, change in LFT results	Smoking and carbamazepine reduce olanzapine levels to a small extent	+++

(Continued)

Table A4.1 (Continued)

Drug	Chemical group	Dose range (daily dose) Single daily dose unless stated (*)	Alternative licensed indications	Adverse effects (See data sheet for full details/ Appendix 6 for comparison)	Interactions	Cost
Quetiapine	Dibenzothiazepine	150–750 mg (*bd) Lower doses in the elderly	None	Hypotension, sedation, dry mouth, constipation, weight gain, dizziness, LFT and TFT changes	Caution with potent inhibitors of CYP3A4, e.g. ketoconazole or nefazodone	+++
Amisulpride	Substituted benzamide	Positive symptoms: 400–1200 mg (*bd) Negative symptoms: 50–300 mg	None	Insomnia, agitation, anxiety, weight gain, extrapyramidal adverse effects, hyperprolactinaemia, sedation	Few known interactions. Caution with other sedatives, including alcohol; dopamine agonists; possibly hypotensive	+++

Ziprasidone	Benzothiazolylpiperazine	40–160 mg (*bd)	Not yet available in UK	Somnolence, nausea. Rarely: dystonia, postural hypotension	Few known interactions. Does not inhibit cytochrome enzymes. Ziprasidone levels slightly decreased by carbamazepine and increased by cimetidine	+++
Zotepine	Dibenzothiepine	50–300 mg (*tds)	None	As for chlorpromazine, + creatinine increase; hypouricaemia	As for chlorpromazine + zotepine levels are increased by CYP3A4 inhibitors, such as diazepam and fluoxetine	++

Appendix 5
Antipsychotic depot injections: suggested dosages and frequencies

Table A5.1 Antipsychotic depot injections: suggested dosages and frequencies

Drug	Trade name	Test dose (mg)	Dose range (mg per week)	Dosing interval (weeks)	Comments
Flupenthixol decanoate	Depixol	20	12.5–400	2–4	Mood elevating; may worsen agitation
Fluphenazine decanoate	Modecate	12.5	6.25–50	2–5	Avoid in depression. High EPSE
Haloperidol decanoate	Haldol	25[a]	12.5–75	4	High EPSE. low incidence of sedation
Pipothiazine palmitate	Piportil Depot	25	12.5–50	4	Lower incidence incidence of EPSE
Zuclopenthixol decanoate	Clopixol	100	100–600	2–4	Useful in agitation and aggression

· Give one-quarter or one-half the stated dosage in the elderly.

· After test dose, wait 4–10 days before starting titration to maintenance therapy.

· Dose range is given in milligrams per week for convenience only; avoid using shorter dosage intervals than those recommended except in exceptional circumstances, for example, if a long interval necessitates a high-volume (> 3–4 mL) injection.

· EPSE, extrapyramidal side-effects.

[a] Test dose not stated by manufacturer.

Appendix 6
Equivalent doses, maximum daily doses, and adverse effects of antipsychotics

Table A6.1 Equivalent doses of antipsychotics

Drug	Equivalent dose (consensus) (mg/day)	Range of values in literature (mg/day)
Chlorpromazine	100	–
Thioridazine	100	75–100
Fluphenazine	2	2–5
Trifluoperazine	5	2.5–5
Flupenthixol	3	2–3
Zuclopenthixol	25	25–60
Haloperidol	3	1.5–5
Droperidol	4	1–4
Sulpiride	200	200–270
Pimozide	2	2
Loxapine	10	10–25
Clozapine	50	50–90
Risperidone	1	0.5–2
Fluphenazine depot	5 (per week)	1–12.5 (per week)
Pipothiazine depot	10 (per week)	10–12.5 (per week)
Flupenthixol depot	10 (per week)	10–20 (per week)
Zuclopenthixol depot	100 (per week)	40–100 (per week)
Haloperidol depot	15 (per week)	5–25 (per week)

All values should be regarded as approximate.

Table A6.2 Oral/parenteral dose equivalents

Drug	Oral dose (mg)	Equivalent IM or IV dose (mg)
Benzodiazepines		
Diazepam	10	10
Lorazepam	4	4
Antipsychotics		
Chlorpromazine	100	25–50
Droperidol	10	7.5
Haloperidol	10	5
Promazine	200	200
Anticholinergics		
Procyclidine	10	7.5

Because of the variation in bioavailability with some drugs, prescriptions should always specify the dose **and** a single route of administration.

Table A6.3 Maximum daily doses of antipsychotics

Drug	Maximum dose (mg/day)
Chlorpromazine	1000
Thioridazine	800
Fluphenazine	20
Trifluoperazine	None
Flupenthixol	18
Zuclopenthixol	150
Haloperidol	30
Sulpiride	2400
Pimozide	20
Loxapine	250
Clozapine	900
Risperidone	16
Fluphenazine depot	50 (per week)
Pipothiazine depot	50 (per week)
Haloperidol depot	300 (every 4 weeks)
Flupenthixol depot	400 (per week)
Zuclopenthixol depot	600 (per week)
Amisulpride	1200
Olanzapine	20
Zotepine	300
Ziprasidone	160
Quetiapine	750

Dosages above these maxima should be used only in extreme circumstances; there is no evidence for improved efficacy. Always follow Royal College of Physicians guidelines.

Table A6.4 Relative adverse effects of antipsychotics

Drug	Sedation	Extrapyramidal	Anticholinergic	Hypotension	Cardiac toxicity
Chlorpromazine	+++	++	++	+++	++
Thioridazine	+++	+	+++	+++	+
Promazine	+++	+	++	++	+
Fluphenazine	+	+++	++	+	+
Perphenazine	+	+++	+	+	+
Trifluoperazine	+	+++	–	+	+
Flupenthixol	+	++	++	+	+
Zuclopenthixol	++	++	++	+	+
Haloperidol	+	+++	+	+	+
Droperidol	++	+++	+	+	+++
Benperidol	+	+++	+	+	+
Sulpiride	–	+	+/–	–	–
Loxapine	++	+++	+	++	+
Clozapine	+++	–	+++	+++	+
Risperidone[a]	+	+	+	+	+
Sertindole	–	–	–	+++	+++
Olanzapine	++	+/–	+	+	–
Quetiapine	++	–	+	++	–
Amisulpride	–	+	–	–	–
Zotepine	+++	++	+	++	++
Ziprasidone	+	+/–	–	+	+

+++, High incidence/severity; ++, moderate; +, low; –, very low/none.
[a]Akathisia common with risperidone.

Appendix 7
Clozapine: management of adverse effects

Table A7.1 Clozapine: management of adverse effects

Adverse effect	Time course	Action
Sedation	First 4 weeks. May persist, but usually wears off	Give smaller dose in the mornings. Some patients can only cope with single night-time dosing. Reduce dose if necessary
Hypersalivation	First 4 weeks. May persist, but usually wears off. Often very troublesome at night	Give hyoscine 300 µg (Kwells) chewed and swallowed at night. Propantheline 15 mg tds may be used but worsens anticholinergic effects. Pirenzepine may be tried. Patients do not always mind excess salivation–treatment not always required
Constipation	Usually persists	Recommend high-fibre diet. Bulk-forming laxatives ± stimulants may be used
Hypotension	First 4 weeks	Advise patient to take time when standing up. Reduce dose or slow down rate of increase. If severe, consider moclobemide and Bovril

(continued)

Table A7.1 (Continued)

Adverse effect	Time course	Action
Tachycardia	First 4 weeks, but often persists	Often occurs if dose escalation is too rapid. Inform patient that it is not dangerous. Give small dose of beta-blocker if necessary
Weight gain	Usually during the first year of treatment	Dietary counselling is essential. Advice may be more effective if given before weight gain occurs. Weight gain is common and often profound (> 2 stones)
Fever	First 3 weeks	Give antipyretic. NB: This fever is not usually related to blood dyscrasias
Seizures	May occur at any time	Dose related. Consider prophylactic valproate[a] if on high dose. After a seizure withhold clozapine for 1 day. Restart at reduced dose. Give sodium valproate
Nausea	First 6 weeks	May give antiemetic. Avoid prochlorperazine and metoclopramide (EPSE)
Neutropenia/ agranulocytosis	First 18 weeks (but may occur at any time)	Stop clozapine; admit to hospital
Nocturnal enuresis	May occur at any time	Try manipulating dose schedule. Avoid fluids before bedtime. In severe cases, desmopressin is usually effective.

[a]Usual dose is 1000–2000 mg/day. Plasma levels may be useful as a rough guide to dosing — aim for 50–100 mg/L. Use of modified–release preparation (Epilim Chrono) may aid compliance: can be given once daily and may be better tolerated.

Index